MCQs in Applied Basic Sciences for Medical Students
Volume 1

Dr Jonathan Fishman &
Dr Laura Fishman

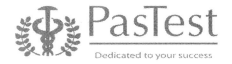

PasTest

Dedicated to your success

MCQs in Applied Basic Sciences for Medical Students
Volume 1

Dr Jonathan Fishman &
Dr Laura Fishman

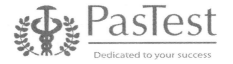

PasTest
Dedicated to your success

© 2006 PASTEST LTD
Egerton Court
Parkgate Estate
Knutsford
Cheshire
WA16 8DX

Telephone: 01565 752000

First Published

ISBN: 1 905635 141
978 1905635 14 6
A catalogue record for this book is available from the British Library.

The information contained within this book was obtained by the author from reliable sources. However, while every effort has been made to ensure its accuracy, no responsibility for loss, damage or injury occasioned to any person acting or refraining from action as a result of information contained herein can be accepted by the publishers or author.

PasTest Revision Books and Intensive Courses

PasTest has been established in the field of postgraduate medical education since 1972, providing revision books and intensive study courses for doctors preparing for their professional examinations.

Books and courses are available for the following specialties:

MRCGP, MRCP Parts 1 and 2, MRCPCH Parts 1 and 2, MRCPsych, MRCS, MRCOG Parts 1 and 2, DRCOG, DCH, FRCA, PLAB Parts 1 and 2.

For further details contact:

PasTest, Freepost, Knutsford, Cheshire WA16 7BR

Tel: 01565 752000 Fax: 01565 650264

www.pastest.co.uk enquiries@pastest.co.uk

Text prepared by Carnegie Book Production, Lancaster
Printed and bound in the UK by Athenaeum Press, Gateshead

Contents

About the authors   vii

Preface   ix

Mastering MCQs   xi

Abbreviations   xiii

Section A

Applied Anatomy   1

    Embryology   3

    Head, neck and spine   9

    Thorax   17

    Abdomen and pelvis   23

    Upper and lower limbs   35

    Section A – Answers   41

Section B

Applied Physiology   141

    Nerve, muscle and neuroscience   143

    Cardiovascular physiology   149

    Respiratory physiology   155

    Renal physiology   161

    Gastrointestinal physiology   167

    Endocrine physiology and thermoregulation   173

    Section B – Answers   181

    Index   258

About the Authors

Dr Jonathan M Fishman, BM BCh (Oxon), MA (Cantab), studied pre-clinical medicine at Sidney Sussex College, University of Cambridge, graduating in 2001 with a first class honours degree in Natural Sciences. He continued with and completed his clinical training at St John's College, Oxford and the John Radcliffe Hospital, qualifying in 2004. He is currently undertaking basic surgical training in London and his interests lie in teaching and medical education.

Dr Laura M Fishman, MB BS, BSc (Hons), is the twin sister of Jonathan Fishman. She qualifed in 2004 from Imperial College London with a first class honours BSc in Endocrinology. She is currently undertaking general medical training in London. She is keen to pursue a career in medicine and maintain an interest in undergraduate education.

Preface

More and more emphasis is being placed on multiple choice questions (MCQs) in the assessment of the medical school curriculum. The reasons for this are several-fold: MCQs have the inherent advantage of being objective and unbiased, in addition to being comparatively easy to mark compared with conventional methods of assessment, such as short answer questions and essay writing. The rapid expansion in both the number of medical schools and the intake of students has led to MCQs becoming the assessment method of choice.

There are many MCQ books currently available. However, there is clearly a need for a MCQ series that deals with the 'early' or 'pre-clinical' years where the emphasis is on the applied basic sciences. A thorough grounding in the basic sciences is necessary, in order successfully to progress through the clinical school years. Indeed the importance of the basic sciences is highlighted by the emphasis placed on these in many of the postgraduate membership examinations that follow.

We have decided to dedicate an entire two volumes of MCQs to the applied basic sciences. This is not because we feel that the applied basic sciences are badly taught (although this may be the case in some medical schools!), but rather because we feel that many young medical students fail to appreciate the significance of learning about particular topics, or fail to make a link between the basic sciences and clinical practice.

The rationale behind this book is not only to provide practice in answering MCQs in the applied basic sciences, but also to bridge the gap between the applied basic sciences and clinical practice. Wherever possible we have endeavoured to correlate the basic sciences with clinical medicine. Not only should this make the basic sciences more enjoyable and retainable, but it will also help the young medical student to recognise and appreciate the importance of learning such material. If after working through these volumes medical students are better able to apply their basic scientific knowledge to clinical practice, we have successfully achieved our goal.

Jonathan Fishman and Laura Fishman

Mastering MCQs

The secret to passing any kind of MCQ exam is to practise as many questions as possible. Sitting in front of large textbooks will help to a degree, but it is important to get a feel for the type of questions that may appear in the exam, and then to focus revision on reading around the questions. Whatever curriculum you currently follow, there will always be core questions that will be tested at the undergraduate level. We hope to cover those core questions.

Each question has five possible answers. One answer will be correct and the other four will be false (single best answer format). One of the first techniques in approaching these types of questions is to cover up the answers initially, read the question and suggest an answer. Then look for the answer in the options available. If the answer appears, you have a very high chance of being correct. You should check that the other answers are in fact incorrect, before selecting your final answer. If you are unable to answer the question initially, work your way down the list and start by eliminating those answers that you definitely feel are incorrect. Even if you are left with two possible answers you have a 50% chance of getting the correct answer by guessing, rather than the 20% chance that you started with. The exam is not usually negatively marked at the undergraduate level, so do not leave or miss out any questions.

If there are any questions that you are unsure of, asterisk that question so that, if you have time, you can come back to it at the end. You should also consider that certain words in the question can give you a clue to getting to the right answer in the exam, eg:

- **'Always'** is, more often than not, **always** false in medicine.
- If the word **'never'** appears, it is always **never** true.

Research has shown that changing your answer in the exam is neither good nor bad: if you have a good reason for changing your answer, then change it. It is a myth that people always change from 'right' to 'wrong', in that it is those questions that you will remember and review after the exam. You will not remember the questions you changed from wrong to right!

Although everyone may tell you before the exam **'READ THE QUESTION'**, it is imperative to do so in the MCQ exam. Underline the key words, and do not be caught out, as people so often are, when the question says which of the following is false as opposed to being true! When you have finished the exam, make a final check that you have answered ALL the questions. Never forget to always ensure that you have answered the last question and not forgotten to turn over to the last page.

We hope you enjoy the book and find it a pleasurable form of learning. All that is left to say is – good luck!

Abbreviations

ABP	arterial blood pressure
ACE	angiotensin-converting enzyme
ACTH	adrenocorticotrophic hormone
ADH	antidiuretic hormone
AMH	anti-Müllerian hormone
ATP	adenosine triphosphate
AV	atrioventricular
Ca^{2+}	calcium ions
cAMP	cyclic AMP
CBF	cerebral blood flow
cGMP	cyclic GMP
Cl^-	chloride
CO	cardiac output
CO	carbon monoxide
CO_2	carbon dioxide
CPP	cerebral perfusion pressure
CRH	corticotrophin-releasing hormone
CSF	cerebrospinal fluid
2,3-DPG	2,3-diphosphoglycerate
DM	diabetes mellitus
ECG	electrocardiogram
Fe^{2+}	ferrous iron
Fe^{3+}	ferric iron
FSH	follicle-stimulating hormone
GFR	glomerular filtration rate
GH	growth hormone
GnRH	gonadotrophin-releasing hormone
H^+	hydrogen ions
H_2O	water

HCO_3^-	bicarbonate
Hb	haemoglobin
HCl	hydrochloric acid
HLA	human leukocyte antigen
HR	heart rate
ICP	intracranial pressure
Ig	immunoglobulin
IVC	inferior vena cava
K^+	potassium ions
LH	luteinising hormone
MABP	mean arterial blood pressure
Na^+	sodium ions
NaCl	sodium chloride
NMJ	neuromuscular junction
$P(O_2)$	partial pressure of oxygen
$P(CO_2)$	partial pressure of carbon dioxide
PAH	p-aminohippuric acid
pH	$-\log_{10}[H^+]$
PTH	parathyroid hormone
PTHrP	parathyroid hormone-related protein
SA	sinoatrial
SV	stroke volume
SVC	superior vena cava
T_3	tri-iodothyronine
T_4	thyroxine
TPR	total peripheral resistance
TRH	thyrotrophin-releasing hormone
TSH	thyroid-stimulating hormone

SECTION A

Applied Anatomy

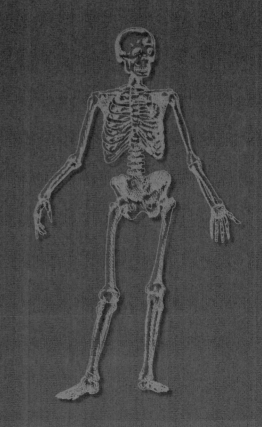

Embryology Questions

1 ▸ The following changes occur at birth:

○ A The left umbilical vein becomes the ligamentum venosum

○ B The urachus becomes the medial umbilical ligament

○ C The ligamentum arteriosum is a remnant of the umbilical arteries

○ D The foramen ovale closes in all cases at birth

○ E The vitellointestinal duct may persist as Meckel's diverticulum

2 ▸ With regard to genital development:

○ A The mesonephric (Wolffian) ducts differentiate into the female genitalia

○ B Female development is hormonally regulated through the actions of anti-Müllerian hormone and testosterone

○ C Gender is principally determined by the presence or absence of two X chromosomes

○ D Anti-Müllerian hormone is secreted by the Leydig cells

○ E The testes and ovaries descend from their original position at the tenth thoracic level

3 ▶ With regard to development of the limbs:

○ A Development occurs in the second trimester of pregnancy

○ B Shaping of the hands and feet is brought about through apoptosis

○ C Development is independent of the apical ectodermal ridge

○ D Thalidomide most commonly causes clinodactyly

○ E Under some circumstances limb regeneration occurs to a small degree in adult humans after amputation

4 ▶ With regard to development of the kidney:

○ A Kidney is derived from endoderm

○ B The transcription factor WT-1 is necessary for induction of the mesenchyme's competence

○ C There are two phases of kidney development

○ D The kidneys descend during development to their final site

○ E The metanephric blastema gives rise to the collecting ducts

5 ▶ With regard to diaphragmatic development:

○ A It is formed by the fusion of two separate elements

○ B It develops in the thoracic region

○ C The left pleuroperitoneal canal is larger and closes later compared with the right

○ D The central tendon arises from the pleuroperitoneal membranes

○ E The septum transversum migrates cranially (rostrally) in development

6 ▶ In craniofacial development:

○ A The human face forms from the fusion of four swellings

○ B Alcohol is the most common cause of holoprosencephaly

○ C The palate forms from the medial extensions of the mandibular swellings

○ D Craniofacial abnormalities account for 5% of all human congenital defects

○ E The nasolacrimal groove forms between the medial and lateral nasal processes

7 In intestinal development:

- ⚪ A The gut is a mesodermal derivative
- ⚪ B The whole of the foregut apart from the stomach undergoes rotation
- ⚪ C The stomach is a midgut derivative
- ⚪ D Rupture of the cloacal membrane creates the mouth
- ⚪ E Midgut development involves herniation of bowel into the umbilicus

8 In the branchial arches:

- ⚪ A Apart from the first cleft, the other branchial clefts are normally obliterated by overgrowth of the second branchial arch
- ⚪ B Six pairs of branchial arches develop in humans
- ⚪ C The muscles of facial expression are derivatives of the first arch
- ⚪ D All parathyroid glands originate from the same branchial arch
- ⚪ E The tongue principally develops from the second branchial arch

9 ▶ Development of the nervous system:

○ A Neural tube development requires signals from the underlying mesoderm

○ B The nervous system is derived from endoderm

○ C Neural tube defects originate during the final trimester of pregnancy

○ D The notochord forms the spinal cord in adults

○ E Neural tube defects result from the incomplete migration of neural crest cells

10 ▶ Meckel's diverticulum:

○ A Is a remnant of the urachus

○ B Is found in 10% of the population

○ C Is most commonly situated immediately adjacent to the vermiform appendix

○ D Is completely asymptomatic and an incidental finding

○ E May contain ectopic tissue

Head, neck and spine
Questions

11 Which of the following cranial nerves carries parasympathetic fibres?

- ○ A V
- ○ B IV
- ○ C VI
- ○ D III
- ○ E II

12 Which of the following is true with regard to the larynx?

- ○ A The posterior cricoarytenoids are the only muscles that separate the vocal folds
- ○ B All the intrinsic muscles are supplied by the recurrent laryngeal nerve
- ○ C The vocal folds are lined by pseudostratified, columnar, ciliated ('respiratory') epithelium
- ○ D The epiglottis is composed largely of hyaline cartilage
- ○ E The cricoid cartilage and tracheal rings are complete rings of cartilage

Answers on page 55

13 With regard to the thyroid gland, which of the following is correct?

○ A The blood supply is through the internal carotid and subclavian arteries

○ B Embryologically the thyroid gland starts at the foramen caecum of the tongue

○ C Venous drainage is by way of the external jugular vein

○ D The thyroid gland produces thyroid-stimulating hormone (TSH)

○ E It is attached to the thyroid cartilage by Berry's ligament

14 With regard to the tongue:

○ A All muscles of the tongue are innervated via the hypoglossal nerve

○ B Special taste sensation on the anterior two-thirds of the tongue is through the mandibular division of the trigeminal nerve

○ C It is composed of smooth musculature

○ D The genioglossus muscle causes the tongue to protrude

○ E Its epithelium is composed of the glandular columnar variety of cells

15 ▶ The parathyroid glands:

○ A Secrete calcitonin
○ B Are always four in number
○ C Are third branchial pouch derivatives
○ D Are all supplied by the inferior thyroid artery
○ E Have an invariable position in the neck

16 ▶ With regard to the extraocular muscles:

○ A Superior rectus is supplied by the trochlear nerve
○ B Levator palpebrae superioris is supplied solely by the oculomotor nerve
○ C The superior oblique muscle is innervated by the oculomotor nerve
○ D Lateral rectus is supplied by the abducens nerve
○ E The inferior oblique muscle moves the eye inferiorly

17 ▶ The palatine tonsil:

○ A Lies on the middle pharyngeal constrictor muscle

○ B Is supplied by the superior pharyngeal artery

○ C Is lined by columnar epithelium

○ D May cause referred pain to the ear if inflamed

○ E After tonsillectomy, can bleed usually as a result of arterial bleeding

18 ▶ The spinal accessory nerve supplies which of the following muscles?

○ A Buccinator

○ B Latissimus dorsi

○ C Trapezius

○ D Stylopharyngeus

○ E Palatoglossus

19 ▶ The parotid gland:

○ A Contains within it, branches of the facial nerve deep to the retromandibular vein

○ B Consists of superficial, middle and deep lobes

○ C Has secretomotor action via the glossopharyngeal and auriculotemporal nerves

○ D Has a duct that pierces the masseter muscle to enter the mouth opposite the upper second molar tooth

○ E Produces mainly a mucus secretion

20 ▶ The cavernous sinus:

○ A Contains the external carotid artery

○ B Lies within the anterior cranial fossa

○ C Contains the pituitary and sphenoidal air sinus within its medial wall

○ D Has blood flow from anterior to posterior via valves

○ E Contains the optic nerve

21 Which of the following muscles is not a muscle of mastication?

○ A Medial pterygoid
○ B Buccinator
○ C Masseter
○ D Lateral pterygoid
○ E Temporalis

22 With regard to the circle of Willis (circulus arteriosus):

○ A It is formed from the anastomosis of the internal and external carotid arteries
○ B The anterior communicating artery joins the two anterior cerebral arteries
○ C The posterior cerebral artery is the terminal branch of the internal carotid artery
○ D The posterior communicating artery joins the two posterior cerebral arteries
○ E The circle of Willis is fascinating, but clinically unimportant

23 With regard to the cranial meninges:

○ A The dura mater is a single layer thick

○ B The pia mater is the outermost layer (closest to the skull)

○ C A subdural haematoma lies in the plane between the dura mater and the arachnoid mater

○ D A subarachnoid haematoma forms on the outside of the dura mater

○ E The dura mater is poorly innervated

24 The facial nerve:

○ A Carries taste sensation from the posterior third of the tongue

○ B Innervates levator palpebrae superioris

○ C Is secretomotor to the lacrimal gland

○ D Is associated with the third branchial arch

○ E Supplies the principal muscles of mastication

With regard to the spinal cord and vertebral column:

○ A The spinal cord terminates at the level of L4

○ B The intervertebral joints are secondary cartilaginous joints

○ C The intervertebral joints are supplied by two anterior spinal arteries and one posterior spinal artery

○ D Batson's vertebral venous plexus contains valves

○ E Intervertebral disc prolapse at L4–5 causes L4 root compression

Thorax
Questions

26 The breast:

- A Drains to the tracheobronchial group of lymph nodes
- B Is supplied mainly by the anterior intercostal arteries
- C Sits on the pectoralis minor muscle
- D Has lymphatics that have connections with those of the opposite breast
- E Involutes during pregnancy

27 With regard to the intercostal spaces:

- A The neurovascular bundle lies between the external intercostal and inner intercostal muscle layers
- B The direction of fibres of the external intercostal muscle is downwards and medial
- C The intercostal vein lies below the intercostal nerve
- D The neurovascular bundle lies in a groove just above each rib
- E The intercostals are the main muscles of respiration

28 With regard to the oesophagus:

○ A It is a segmental muscular tube composed entirely of smooth muscle

○ B The epithelium is always stratified squamous throughout its whole length

○ C The blood supply is from the descending thoracic aorta along its entire length

○ D It lacks a true serosal surface

○ E It measures about 40 cm in length

29 Which of the following is true with regard to oesophageal constrictions?

○ A The lower oesophageal sphincter is a true anatomical sphincter

○ B Oesophageal constrictions may be caused by the right principal bronchus

○ C The narrowest part of the oesophagus is at the level of cricopharyngeus

○ D Oesophageal constrictions may be caused by the normal size of the left atrium

○ E They may be caused by the descending thoracic aorta

30 ▶ The diaphragm:

○ A Is composed of smooth muscle
○ B Contracts with expiration
○ C Forms the main muscle of respiration at rest
○ D Has motor innervation through the right and left phrenic nerves and lower intercostal nerves
○ E Has sensation to the diaphragm through only the lower intercostal nerves

31 ▶ With regard to diaphragmatic openings:

○ A The inferior vena cava passes through the muscular part of the diaphragm at T8
○ B The aortic opening lies at the level of T10
○ C The oesophageal opening transmits the right phrenic nerve
○ D The left phrenic nerve passes with the oesophagus through the oesophageal opening
○ E The sympathetic trunks pass posterior to the medial arcuate ligament

32 ▶ The thoracic duct:

○ A Drains into the confluence of the right internal jugular and subclavian veins

○ B Lies anterior to the oesophagus as it passes through the diaphragm

○ C Crosses the midline at the level of T5

○ D Has no valves

○ E If injured, may result in a haemothorax

33 ▶ With regard to the lungs:

○ A The left lung has three lobes

○ B The horizontal fissure is present in the left lung

○ C Each lung has eight bronchopulmonary segments

○ D A foreign body is more likely to enter the left than the right bronchus

○ E The lungs receive a dual blood supply

34 ▶ With regard to the pleura:

- ○ A The pleura ends level with the twelfth rib posteriorly
- ○ B It extends above the clavicle superiorly
- ○ C The visceral layer is richly innervated
- ○ D It extends above the neck of the first rib superiorly
- ○ E The pleural reflection on the right side is identical to that on the left side

35 ▶ With regard to the pericardium:

- ○ A The pericardium is two layers thick
- ○ B It is poorly innervated
- ○ C It is responsible for the formation of the transverse and oblique sinuses
- ○ D Pericardiocentesis may be detrimental in the management of cardiac tamponade
- ○ E The pericardium is essential in order to maintain a normal cardiac output

36 ▶ Which of the following about the coronary arteries is correct:

○ A The sinoatrial (SA) node is supplied by the left coronary artery in most cases

○ B The atrioventricular (AV) node is supplied by the left coronary artery in most cases

○ C The circumflex artery is a branch of the right coronary artery

○ D Occlusion of the anterior interventricular artery (left anterior descending artery) results in an anterior myocardial infarction

○ E Angina is always caused by atherosclerosis of the coronary vessels

Abdomen and pelvis
Questions

37 Concerning the inguinal canal:

○ A The superficial inguinal ring is a hole in transversalis fascia

○ B The canal runs from the anterosuperior iliac spine to the pubic tubercle

○ C The conjoint tendon is formed by fusion of external and internal oblique muscles

○ D The posterior wall of the canal is bounded by transversalis fascia and the conjoint tendon medially

○ E A direct inguinal hernia passes through both the deep and the superficial inguinal rings

38 Concerning the epiploic foramen (of Winslow), which of the following is true?

○ A The posterior wall is formed from the lesser omentum
○ B The portal vein lies in its posterior wall
○ C The quadrate lobe of the liver lies superiorly
○ D The common bile duct sits in the free edge of the greater omentum anteriorly
○ E The epiploic foramen forms the entrance to the lesser sac

39 Which of the following are features of the small bowel?

○ A Valvulae conniventes
○ B Haustra
○ C Sacculations
○ D Appendices epiploicae
○ E Taeniae coli

40 The gallbladder:

A Has epithelium that is stratified squamous

B Has a normal capacity of around 10 mL

C Is supplied by the cystic artery, a branch of the left hepatic artery

D Is stimulated to contract by cholecystokinin

E Is essential for life

41 With regard to the gallbladder disease:

A Courvoisier's law states that, in the presence of obstructive jaundice, an impalpable gallbladder is always the result of gallstones

B Gallbladder disease may refer pain to the right shoulder tip

C The surface marking of the gallbladder is the right sixth intercostal space, midclavicular line

D Gallstones are usually made up of calcium carbonate

E Gallstones always cause symptoms

42 ▶ With regard to the liver:

○ A It is completely surrounded by peritoneum

○ B The ligamentum venosum is a remnant of the umbilical vein

○ C It receives oxygen from the hepatic artery only

○ D It is surrounded by Gerota's fascia

○ E The right subhepatic space or hepatorenal pouch (of Rutherford–Morison) is the most dependent part of the peritoneal cavity

43 ▶ Portosystemic anastomoses:

○ A Occur at sites at which arterial blood meets venous blood

○ B Feature at the lower end of the oesophagus

○ C Become highly significant in renal failure

○ D Are most clinically significant at the lower end of the anal canal

○ E Feature at the splenic hilum

44 ▶ The spleen:

○ A Lies under cover of the ninth to eleventh ribs on the right

○ B Is the major site of erythropoietin secretion

○ C Is normally the site of haematopoiesis in adults

○ D As an accessory spleen is rare

○ E If removed from a patient leaves him or her at high risk of post-splenectomy sepsis

45 ▶ The transpyloric plane (of Addison):

○ A Is halfway between the suprasternal notch and umbilicus

○ B Lies at the level of T12

○ C Lies at the origin of the inferior mesenteric artery

○ D Lies level with the hilum of the kidneys

○ E Is the point at which the aorta bifurcates

46 With regard to the adrenal gland (suprarenal gland):

○ A The suprarenal vein on each side drains into the corresponding renal vein

○ B The adrenal gland is situated within the same fascial compartment as the kidney

○ C The zona glomerulosa forms the innermost layer of the adrenal cortex

○ D The anterior surface of the right adrenal gland is overlapped by the inferior vena cava

○ E The adrenal medulla is derived from embryonic mesoderm

47 The vermiform appendix:

○ A Is most often situated in a pelvic position

○ B Receives blood via the right colic branch of the superior mesenteric artery

○ C Lies at McBurney's point (halfway between the anterosuperior iliac spine and umbilicus)

○ D Is unimportant in humans

○ E Is a retroperitoneal structure

48 ▶ Acute appendicitis:

○ A Is most common at the extremes of age

○ B Can result in thrombosis of the appendicular artery (endarteritis obliterans)

○ C Often resolves with conservative management such as antibiotics

○ D If untreated, is rarely life threatening

○ E Classically refers pain to the epigastric region

49 ▶ The greater omentum:

○ A Has no surgical importance

○ B Is supplied by the right and left gastric arteries

○ C Is two layers thick

○ D Provides a route of access to the lesser sac

○ E Has anterior layers that descend from the lesser curvature of the stomach

50 ▶ The ureters:

○ A Are lined by stratified squamous epithelium

○ B Enter the bladder obliquely forming a flap valve

○ C Have their point of narrowest calibre at the pelviureteric junction

○ D Have an arterial supply to their lower third by way of the descending abdominal aorta

○ E In females are crossed below by the uterine arteries in the broad ligament

51 ▶ The spermatic cord:

○ A Contains within it the ilioinguinal nerve

○ B Contains the femoral branch of the genitofemoral nerve

○ C Is surrounded by two fascial coverings

○ D Contains the pampiniform plexus

○ E Has dartos muscle contained in its wall

52 ► The testis:

○ A Is supplied by the testicular artery, which arises from the internal iliac artery

○ B Drains bilaterally via the pampiniform plexus to the inferior vena cava

○ C Has lymph drainage to the inguinal group of lymph nodes

○ D Is supplied by T10 sympathetic nerves

○ E A fluid collection around it is known as a varicocele

53 ► The ovary:

○ A Is retroperitoneal

○ B Lies medial to the obturator nerve and anterior to the ureter

○ C Drains lymph to the internal iliac nodes

○ D Receives a parasympathetic supply from the pudendal nerve

○ E Gives rise to referred pain in the suprapubic region

54 ▶ The rectum:

○ A Is drained by tributaries of both the inferior mesenteric and internal iliac veins

○ B Is suspended by a mesentery

○ C Receives its blood supply from the external iliac artery

○ D Is lined by transitional epithelium

○ E Is supplied by parasympathetic nerve fibres from the vagus

55 ▶ With regard to the uterus:

○ A It usually lies in a retroverted, anteflexed position

○ B The broad ligament is a remnant of the gubernaculum

○ C The pouch of Douglas lies between the bladder anteriorly and the uterus posteriorly

○ D The ovarian artery is intimately related to the ureter

○ E The ureter is closely related to the lateral fornix of the cervix

56 ▶ With regard to the blood supply of the stomach:

○ A The right half of the lesser curvature is supplied by the right gastroepiploic artery

○ B The left half of the greater curvature is supplied by the left gastric artery

○ C The fundus of the stomach is supplied by the left gastric artery

○ D The gastroduodenal artery is a branch of the common hepatic artery

○ E The right gastric artery is most commonly implicated in a bleeding duodenal ulcer

Upper and lower limbs

Questions

57 ▶ Concerning the femoral triangle, which of the following is correct?

○ A The femoral vein lies lateral to the femoral artery

○ B The femoral nerve lies within the femoral sheath

○ C The femoral artery lies at the midpoint of the inguinal ligament

○ D The femoral nerve is the most medially placed structure

○ E Cloquet's node lies most medially within the femoral canal

58 ▶ The shoulder (glenohumeral) joint:

○ A Is a ball-and-socket fibrocartilaginous joint

○ B Has high mobility at the expense of stability

○ C Is supported mainly by ligaments

○ D Lies in close relation to the musculocutaneous nerve

○ E Most commonly dislocates posteriorly

59 ► Which of the following is true with regard to the hip joint?

○ A The blood supply to the femoral head arises from a single source

○ B The hip joint can refer pain to the knee

○ C The hip joint is the most commonly dislocated joint in the body

○ D The hip joint lies deep to the sciatic nerve

○ E The fibrous capsule is strengthened by two ligaments

60 ► With regard to the anatomical snuffbox:

○ A Tenderness at its base is indicative of a fractured hamate

○ B It is bounded medially by abductor pollicis longus

○ C The basilic vein begins in its roof

○ D The skin overlying it is supplied by cutaneous branches of the median nerve

○ E The pulsation of the radial artery may be felt at its base

61 With regard to the knee joint:

◯ A It is a synovial, pivot joint

◯ B The cruciate ligaments are intracapsular and intrasynovial

◯ C The suprapatellar bursa (pouch) communicates with the knee joint

◯ D Inflammation of the prepatellar bursa is known as clergyman's knee

◯ E The menisci play an important role in the mechanism of locking and unlocking of the knee joint

62 Which of the following is true with regard to the brachial plexus?

◯ A The brachial plexus has principal root values C6–T2

◯ B The serratus anterior muscle is innervated by the subscapular nerve

◯ C A lesion involving the lower roots of the brachial plexus results in a classic Erb–Duchenne palsy

◯ D Cords lie in relation to the third part of the axillary artery

◯ E Roots lie in the neck between the scalenus anterior and medius muscles

63   With regard to the brachial plexus:

○ A   The ulnar nerve arises from the posterior cord

○ B   The radial nerve arises from the lateral cord

○ C   The musculocutaneous nerve arises from the lateral cord

○ D   The median nerve arises from the anterior cord

○ E   The axillary nerve arises from the lateral cord

64   The carpal tunnel:

○ A   Is a fibro-osseous tunnel containing the extensor tendons

○ B   Contains the ulnar nerve and artery within it

○ C   When it involves entrapment of the median nerve within, it is known as cubital tunnel syndrome

○ D   Contains 10 tendons within it

○ E   Contains the palmar cutaneous branch of the median nerve within it

65 ▶ Concerning the arterial supply of the lower limb:

○ A The femoral artery is a direct continuation of the common iliac artery

○ B The posterior tibial pulse is posterior to the lateral malleolus at the ankle

○ C The popliteal pulse is the most superficial structure within the popliteal fossa

○ D The femoral pulse lies at the mid-point of the inguinal ligament

○ E The dorsalis pedis pulse is lateral to the extensor hallucis longus tendon

66 ▶ With regard to the superficial veins of the extremities:

○ A The cephalic vein lies within the deltopectoral groove

○ B The long (great) saphenous vein lies behind the medial malleolus at the ankle

○ C The short (small) saphenous vein enters the femoral vein

○ D The basilic vein pierces the clavipectoral fascia

○ E The long saphenous vein has no tributaries draining into it

With regard to the hand:

○ A All the lumbricals are supplied by the median nerve
○ B All the interossei are supplied by the ulnar nerve
○ C The palmar interossei abduct the fingers
○ D It is supplied by a single palmar arterial arch
○ E Dupuytren's contracture is caused by ischaemic contracture of the intrinsic muscles of the hand

Embryology
Answers

 1   **E**   The vitellointestinal duct may persist as Meckel's diverticulum

There are many important changes that take place at birth:

- The urachus (allantois) becomes the single median , umbilical ligament.

- The umbilical arteries become the right and left medial umbilical ligaments, respectively.

- The ductus venosus becomes the ligamentum venosum.

- The left umbilical vein becomes the ligamentum teres (round ligament) in the free edge of the falciform ligament.

- The ductus arteriosus becomes the ligamentum arteriosum.

- In 2% of cases the vitellointestinal duct may persist as Meckel's diverticulum.

- The foramen ovale in most cases obliterates at birth to become the fossa ovalis, but remains patent into adulthood in some 20% of cases.

Aberrations of this normal developmental process may lead to problems in adulthood. Failure of the urachus (which normally runs from the bladder to the umbilicus) to obliterate correctly may lead to a urachal fistula, sinus, diverticulum or cyst, often

Embryology – Answers

with leakage of urine from the umbilicus. Failure of the ductus arteriosus to obliterate at birth leads to a patent ductus arteriosus, resulting in non-cyanotic congenital heart disease. In 2% of cases, the vitellointestinal duct persists as Meckel's diverticulum with its associated complications. In some 20% of cases the foramen ovale fails to obliterate completely at birth, resulting in a patent foramen ovale. This may become the site for paradoxical embolism (where venous thrombus migrates and enters the systemic circulation through a patent foramen ovale), resulting in stroke.

2 ▶ E The testes and ovaries descend from their original position at the tenth thoracic level

Genital development is principally determined by the presence or absence of a Y chromosome. Thus, XO individuals (Turner's syndrome) are female and XXY individuals (Klinefelter's syndrome) are male. Presence of the sex-determining region of the Y chromosome (SRY) results in male development; absence of the SRY leads to female development.

If the embryo is male, the *SRY* gene is transcribed and this initiates a cascade of events. The sex cord forms the seminiferous tubules, and some of the support cells become Sertoli cells and produce a hormone known as anti-Müllerian hormone (AMH), whereas other support cells become Leydig cells and secrete testosterone. This has the consequence that the paramesonephric (Müllerian) ducts regress as a result of AMH and the external genitalia become male (conversion of testosterone to dihydrotestosterone in the genital fold results in formation of the penis and scrotum). The mesonephric (Wolffian) ducts grow to form the vas deferens and associated ducts. In females, where there is no *SRY* gene, the support cells do not form Sertoli cells. This has the consequence that no AMH is produced and no testosterone-secreting cells develop. The paramesonephric (Müllerian) ducts remain and form the uterus and fallopian tubes; the mesonephric (Wolffian) ducts regress and female external genitalia develop (labia majora and minora, and clitoris). Aberrations of this process may lead to ambiguous genitalia and problems with gender assignment.

During embryonic and fetal life, the testes and the ovaries both descend from their original position at the tenth thoracic level. This explains the long course taken by the gonadal arteries and the site of referred pain from the gonads to the umbilicus (T10 dermatome). Descent is genetically, hormonally and anatomically regulated and depends on a ligamentous cord known as the gubernaculum. Furthermore, descent of the testis through the inguinal canal into the scrotum depends on an evagination of peritoneum known as the processus vaginalis. This normally obliterates at birth. Gonadal descent is a complicated process and there are therefore many ways in which it can go wrong. Most commonly, an undescended, or maldescended, testis may occur (cryptorchidism). A patent processus vaginalis may lead to the formation of a congenital hydrocele or inguinal hernia.

3   B   Shaping of the hands and feet is brought about through apoptosis

The limb is probably the organ with the best understood development; to understand limb abnormalities it is necessary to understand how the limb develops. Limb development takes places over a 4-week period; by the end of week 8 of development all the components of the upper and lower limbs are distinct. During this critical period, limb development is susceptible to the harmful effects of environmental teratogens, resulting in limb anomalies.

The limbs develop from small protrusions (the limb buds) that arise from the body wall of the embryo. Positioning and patterning the limb involve cellular interactions between the ectoderm surrounding the limb bud (apical ectodermal ridge) and the mesenchymal cells that form the core of the limb bud.

As the limb grows out, the cells acquire a positional value that relates to their position in the bud with respect to all three axes: proximodistal, anteroposterior and dorsoventral. These positional values largely determine how the cells will develop. The positional value of the cells is acquired in the progress zone at the tip of the growing bud. Thalidomide, a commonly used drug in the late 1950s and early 1960s for morning sickness, was later found to interfere with the normal processes of limb development, resulting in major limb defects such as phocomelia (short, ill-formed limbs resembling the flippers of a seal) and amelia (absent limbs). Clinodactyly is associated with Down's syndrome.

Separation of the digits occurs by apoptosis (or programmed cell death). This is a good example of a situation in which apoptosis is physiological, rather than pathological.

Adult human limbs never regenerate after an amputation, under any circumstances. Adult human limb loss is permanent and irreversible. Some amphibians are, however, unique among vertebrates in being able to regenerate entire limbs. This relates to their ability to revert to an embryonic state (dedifferentiate) in order to restart embryogenesis. Elucidation of the mechanisms involved in amphibians, and its possible relationship to limb development in higher organisms, may enable us to regenerate a lost limb after an amputation.

4 **B The transcription factor WT-1 is necessary for induction of the mesenchyme's competence**

The kidney develops from the intermediate column of mesoderm. There are three phases of kidney development; the definitive kidney develops in the last phase:

Stage 1:   pronephros – primitive tubules.

Stage 2:   mesonephros – functional in the embryo, producing a dilute urine that is important in maintaining the composition of the amniotic fluid; also contributes to the male genital system.

Stage 3:   metanephros – true, hind kidneys.

The definitive metanephroi are induced early in week 5 by the ureteric buds, which sprout from the mesonephric ducts. The ureteric bud induces the mesenchymal cells to condense around it, forming the metanephric blastema. The development of the ureteric bud and the metanephric blastema depends on reciprocal induction, neither being able to develop in the absence of the other. The metanephric blastema causes the ureteric bud to grow and bifurcate and the ureteric bud induces the mesenchyme to differentiate into nephrons. If the ureteric bud does not reach, or signal properly to the surrounding mesenchyme, or vice versa, a kidney will not form (renal agenesis). If the ureteric bud bifurcates prematurely, a bifid ureter may result. Alternatively, if two ureteric buds develop, an ectopic ureter may result.

The ureteric bud branches and gives rise to the collecting ducts and ureters; the metanephric blastema gives rise to the tubules, or nephrons.

The transcription factor and tumour suppressor gene, *WT-1*, is expressed in metanephric blastema, making it competent to receive signals from the ureteric bud that are essential for its induction. Mutations in the gene are associated with a cancer of the kidney in children known as Wilms' tumour.

The kidneys ascend from their original sacral location to a lumbar site. The mechanism responsible is not understood, but the differential growth of the lumbar and sacral regions of the embryo may play a role. Several anomalies can arise from variations in this process of ascent. A kidney may fail to ascend, remaining as a pelvic kidney. The inferior poles of the two metanephroi may fuse during ascent, forming a U-shaped horseshoe kidney. During ascent this kidney becomes caught under the inferior mesenteric artery and so does not reach its normal site.

5   C   The left pleuroperitoneal canal is larger and closes later compared with the right

The diaphragm is a composite musculotendinous structure formed in the embryo by the fusion of four separate elements:

1. Septum transversum (giving rise to the non-muscular central tendon).

2. Pleuroperitoneal membranes: closes the primitive communication between the pleural and peritoneal cavities (forms the bulk of the diaphragmatic muscle).

3. A peripheral rim derived from the body wall (paraxial mesoderm).

4. Dorsal oesophageal mesenchyme (forms the left and right crura).

The septum transversum develops within the cervical region. This explains how the diaphragm derives its innervation from the phrenic nerve (C3, C4, C5, keep the diaphragm alive!). Caudal translocation of the septum transversum is accompanied by elongation of the phrenic nerves and explains the long course of the phrenic nerve (from the cervical roots) through the thoracic cavity.

In a congenital diaphragmatic hernia, one of the pleuroperitoneal canals (that forms a communication between the pleural and peritoneal cavities, respectively) fails to close off through failure of pleuroperitoneal membrane development. This allows the developing abdominal viscera to bulge into the pleural cavity. If the mass of displaced viscera is large enough, it will stunt the growth of lung on that side, resulting in pulmonary hypoplasia and respiratory insufficiency, which may be fatal. The left side is involved four to eight times more often than the right, primarily because the left pleuroperitoneal canal is larger and closes later than the right, but also because of the liver on the right side.

6   B   Alcohol is the most common cause of holoprosencephaly

The human face forms from the fusion of five facial swellings:

- median frontonasal prominence (in front of forebrain)
- bilateral maxillary swellings (first arch derivative)
- bilateral mandibular swellings (first arch derivative).

All appear by the end of week 4 of development.

In week 5 of development, a pair of ectodermal thickenings appears on the frontonasal process, called the nasal placode. In week 6, the nasal placode divides into medial and lateral nasal processes. The groove between the lateral nasal process and the adjacent maxillary swelling is called the nasolacrimal groove. This later forms the nasolacrimal duct, which drains excess tears from the conjunctiva of the eye into the inferior meatus of the nasal cavity. The palate forms from medial extensions of the maxillary swellings, the palatine shelves, which fuse with each other in the midline. An appreciation of the five facial swellings helps to explain how the different parts of the face are innervated separately via the different branches of the trigeminal nerve.

In this remodelling process all the different parts must be in register to ensure perfect fusion. This is complex, both temporally and spatially, so craniofacial development is highly sensitive to perturbations. Indeed craniofacial abnormalities account for a third of all human congenital defects. Anomalies in the fusion of the five facial swellings result in facial clefts, eg cleft lip results when the maxillary swelling fails to fuse correctly with the medial nasal process and cleft palate results from incomplete fusion of the palatine shelves. These clefts can be of variable severity, are sometimes bilateral and have a number of causes.

The term 'holoprosencephaly' refers to a spectrum of malformations of the head midline, including abnormal development of the forebrain, medial nasal processes and associated midfacial structures (eg nasal bones and septum). In severe cases this may result in a single nostril (cebocephalia) with close-set eyes (hypotelorism) or even a single eye (cyclopia). It is most commonly caused by alcohol consumption during the first month of pregnancy, being the most disabling manifestation of fetal alcohol syndrome. Alcohol is now regarded as the most common cause of congenital mental handicap in the western world.

E Midgut development involves herniation of bowel into the umbilicus

The gut is an endodermal derivative created from a midline gut tube through a complex series of rotations.

The gut is divided into three distinct territories:

1. Foregut: mouth up to second part of duodenum

2. Midgut: second part of duodenum up to two-thirds of the way along the transverse colon

3. Hindgut: two-thirds of the way along the transverse colon up to the anus.

This distinction is important developmentally, anatomically and clinically

One consequence of the midline development of the gut is that visceral pain arising from the intestine often refers to the midline in the adult. Thus, foregut pain typically refers to the epigastric region, midgut pain to the periumbilical region and hindgut pain to the suprapubic region.

The cranial end of the embryological gut tube is capped by the buccopharyngeal membrane and the caudal end by the cloacal membrane. Both later rupture, forming the orifices of the body (ie the mouth and anus, respectively).

The stomach forms the thoracic part of the foregut. The dorsal wall of the stomach grows faster than the ventral wall, resulting in a dorsal 'greater curvature' and a ventral 'lesser curvature'. Subsequently the stomach rotates 90° about the craniocaudal axis. As a result the greater curvature lies to the left. This has the consequence that the two vagus nerves that initially flanked the stomach on the left and right now lie posterior and anterior in the region of the stomach (remembered by the mnemonic RIP, or right is posterior). An additional tilting caudally orients the greater curvature so that it lies inferiorly.

Excessive growth of the midgut results in its herniation into the umbilicus, forming the primary intestinal loop. This loop undergoes a 90° rotation anti-clockwise. Subsequently the midgut is rapidly retracted into the abdomen and, as it does so, it rotates anti-clockwise a further 180°. Finally the caecum moves inferiorly to give the definitive organisation of the intestine. If the anterior abdominal wall does not close completely, loops of midgut may remain outside the abdominal cavity at birth forming a condition known as omphalocele or gastroschisis. Abnormal rotation of gut can cause a spectrum of anomalies, eg there may be freely (malrotated) suspended coils of intestine that are prone to volvulus, causing constriction of its blood supply.

8   A   Apart from the first cleft, the other bronchial clefts are normally obliterated by overgrowth of the second branchial arch

The pharyngeal, or branchial, arches are the mammalian equivalent of the gill arches in fish. In humans, there are five pairs of branchial arches, which develop in a craniocaudal sequence (equivalent to gill arches 1, 2, 3, 4 and 6).

Note that the fifth branchial arch never forms in humans, or forms as a short-lived rudiment and promptly regresses. Each arch contains a central cartilaginous element, striated muscle, cranial nerve and aortic arch artery, surrounded by ectoderm on the outside and lined by endoderm. The arches are separated externally by ectodermally lined branchial clefts and internally by endodermally lined branchial pouches:

- First arch gives muscles of mastication.

- Second arch gives muscles of facial expression.
- Third and fourth arches give muscles of vocalisation and deglutition.
- Sixth arch gives the intrinsic muscles of the larynx.

Certain key features concerning the branchial arches are worth remembering:

- The superior parathyroid glands develop from the fourth branchial pouch; the inferior parathyroids, along with the thymus, are third pouch derivatives. Consequently, the inferior parathyroids may migrate with the thymus down into the mediastinum, and hence its liability to end up in unusual positions.

- The tongue is derived from several sources. The anterior two-thirds of the tongue mucosa is a first arch derivative, whereas the posterior third is contributed to by the third and fourth arches. The tongue muscles, in contrast, are formed from occipital somite mesoderm. For this reason, the motor and sensory nerve fibres of the tongue are carried by separate sets of cranial nerves.

- The thyroid gland arises from between the first and second arches as a diverticulum (thyroglossal duct), which grows downwards leaving the foramen caecum at its origin. Incomplete thyroid descent may give rise to a lingual thyroid or a thyroglossal cyst.

- Apart from the first branchial cleft (which forms the external ear), the other clefts are normally obliterated by overgrowth of the second pharyngeal arch, enclosing the remaining clefts in a transient, ectoderm-lined, lateral cervical sinus. This space normally disappears rapidly and completely. It may persist in adulthood as a branchial cyst or fistula.

9   **A**   Neural tube development requires signals from the underlying mesoderm

The nervous system arises from a special type of ectoderm that has been neurally induced to form neuroectoderm. The first stage in neurulation (ie development of the nervous system) is the establishment in the ectoderm of a region of cells that acquire neural competence (neural induction). The second stage is the morphogenetic process of neurulation, which transforms the neuroepithelial sheet into the neural tube.

Neurulation involves communication between the mesoderm and the overlying ectoderm. The mesoderm primarily involved is the notochord, a dense rod of axial mesoderm that is very important in patterning the embryo early in development, but forms only the nucleus pulposus in the adult (in the centre of the intervertebral disc) and the apical ligament of the dens. Signals (specialised secreted proteins) are secreted by the notochord and induce the specialisation of the overlying ectoderm cells to form the floor of the neural tube.

Closure of the neural tube proceeds bidirectionally, ending with closure of the cranial and caudal openings (neuropores). The cranial neuropore finally closes on day 24 and the caudal neuropore on day 26 of development. Closure of the neural tube is susceptible and a common cause of birth defects.

The neural crest, a migratory cell population, begins to emigrate from the dorsal half of the neural tube around the time of neural tube closure. It has a diverse and complex fate that includes cartilage in the head, melanocytes, the medullary cells of the adrenal gland, glial Schwann cells, and neurons of both the peripheral and autonomic nervous systems. Aberrant neural crest migration may result in Hirschsprung's disease of the bowel (congenital megacolon or aganglionosis), but not neural tube defects.

A variety of malformations result from failure of part of the neural tube and overlying skeleton to close, usually at the cranial or caudal end of the nervous system. Such neural tube defects originate during the third week of development and are the most common group of neurological malformations encountered in humans, occurring in 1 in 300–5000 births, depending on the geographical region. In spina bifida, the vertebral arch is defective dorsally, usually caudally in the lumbrosacral region (termed spina bifida occulta in its mild form), and in severe cases the meninges protrudes from the vertebral canal (meningocele), sometimes including neural tissue (myelomeningocele) with associated neural impairment. Rarely, failure of cranial neural tube closure results in anencephaly where the forebrain is in contact with the amniotic fluid and degenerates (it is fatal). About 50% of neural tube defects may be prevented by women taking folic acid, even in the babies of mothers who have previously given birth to infants with neural tube defects. However, it must be taken during the first few weeks of pregnancy because this is when the neural tube is closing and hence susceptible to perturbations.

10   E   May contain ectopic tissue

Meckel's diverticulum is the anatomical remnant of the vitellointestinal duct, which, in the developing fetus, connects the primitive midgut to the yolk sac and also plays a part in intestinal rotation. The urachus (a derivative of the allantois) is different and connects the bladder to the umbilicus in the fetus. After birth the urachus becomes known as the median umbilical ligament.

The vitellointestinal duct normally regresses between weeks 5 and 8 of development, but in 2% of individuals it persists as a remnant of variable length and location, known as Meckel's diverticulum, in honour of JF Meckel who first discussed the embryological basis of this anomaly in the nineteenth century. Most often it is observed as a 5-cm (2-inch) intestinal diverticulum projecting from the anti-mesenteric wall of the ileum, about 60 cm (2 feet) from the ileocaecal valve. It is about twice as common in males as in females. However, this useful mnemonic ('the rule of 2s') holds true only in two-thirds of cases; the length of the diverticulum is variable and its site may be more proximal.

It is estimated that 15–30% of individuals with Meckel's diverticulum develop symptoms from intestinal obstruction, gastrointestinal bleeding, acute inflammation (diverticulitis) or perforation. Its blind end may contain ectopic tissue, namely gastric mucosa (in 10% cases), liver, pancreatic tissue, or carcinoid or lymphoid tissue. This is important because gastric mucosa bears HCl-secreting parietal cells and can therefore ulcerate within the diverticulum (similar to a stomach ulcer), causing bleeding. Bowel obstruction may result from the trapping of part of the small bowel by a fibrous band (which represents a remnant of the vitelline vessels), connecting the diverticulum to the umbilicus. Symptoms may closely mimic appendicitis. Therefore, if a normal-looking appendix is found at laparoscopy, or during an open appendicectomy, it is important to exclude Meckel's diverticulum as a cause of the patient's symptoms. The mortality rate in untreated cases is estimated to be 2.5–15%.

Head, neck and spine
Answers

 11 ▶ D III

There are 12 pairs of cranial nerves that, together with the 31 pairs of spinal nerves, constitute the peripheral nervous system. The central nervous system comprises the brain and spinal cord.

A peripheral nerve is a mixed nerve containing motor, sensory and autonomic (parasympathetic, sympathetic) elements. Parasympathetic outflow arises from the 'craniosacral' region, ie from certain cranial nerves and sacral roots S2–4. Cranial nerves III (oculomotor), VII (facial), IX (glossopharyngeal) and X (vagus) carry parasympathetic fibres with functions that are primarily secretomotor (eg salivary secretions in the case of cranial nerve VII) and ciliary motor (pupillary reflexes and accommodation in the case of cranial nerve III), whereas cranial nerves IX and X play an integral role in blood pressure regulation. Sympathetic outflow is principally 'thoracolumbar' (ie from spinal segments T1 to L2). The sympathetic nervous system has vasomotor (vascular tone), sudomotor (sweating) and pilomotor functions, in addition to controlling smooth muscle and sphincter tone, and playing a key role in cardiovascular homoeostasis.

Understanding the above makes it easy to predict the outcome of particular lesions in certain clinical settings. Take an oculomotor (III) cranial nerve palsy, for instance. Interruption of the parasympathetic fibres to the constrictor pupillae muscle results in a unilaterally dilated pupil (mydriasis) as an important hallmark of a third nerve palsy. This characteristic can thus easily be distinguished from Horner's syndrome (sympathetic chain disruption), which causes a unilaterally constricted pupil (miosis).

12   A   The posterior cricoarytenoids are the only muscles that separate the vocal folds

The posterior cricoarytenoid muscles are perhaps the most important muscles in the body because they are the only intrinsic muscles of the larynx that open up the airway by separating the vocal folds. Without them asphyxiation would quickly ensue.

All the intrinsic muscles of the larynx are supplied by the recurrent laryngeal nerve of the vagus, with the exception of the important cricothyroid muscle, which is supplied by the external branch of the superior laryngeal nerve. The cricothyroid is the muscle that is principally concerned with altering voice pitch by altering the length of the vocal folds. Damage to the superior laryngeal or recurrent laryngeal nerves can occur during thyroid, oesophageal or aortic arch surgery, leading to changes in the character of the voice and even airway compromise (Semon's law).

The true vocal folds form the superior border of the cricothyroid membrane and are lined by stratified squamous mucosa, not the typical respiratory epithelium that lines the rest of the respiratory tract. This confers protective properties on the vocal folds, which are subject to 'wear and tear' from vocalisation. The same is true of the epiglottis, which is also lined by 'protective' stratified squamous epithelium. It is largely composed of elastic cartilage, rather than hyaline cartilage.

The cricoid cartilage is the only complete ring of cartilage within the human body, in contrast to the tracheal rings, which are C-shaped rings of hyaline cartilage that provide support to the trachea but are deficient posteriorly.

13   B   Embryologically the thyroid gland starts at the foramen caecum of the tongue

The thyroid gland is an endocrine gland that sits at the base of the neck like a bow tie. It consists of two lateral lobes and an isthmus, which is attached via Berry's ligament to the second to fourth tracheal rings (it is not attached to the thyroid cartilage, but sits lower down in the neck). The fact that the thyroid gland is attached to the trachea by Berry's ligament, and also that it is invested within pretracheal fascia, explains why the thyroid gland moves up with swallowing. This is important clinically because it defines a swelling within the neck as being of thyroid origin.

The embryology is important. The thyroid gland descends from the foramen caecum which lies between the anterior two-thirds and posterior third of the tongue via the thyroglossal duct. If the embryology goes wrong it can lead to problems in later adult life. An incompletely descended thyroid gland may persist in adult life as a lingual thyroid or thyroglossal cyst.

The blood supply to the thyroid is by way of the superior thyroid artery (a branch of the external thyroid artery), the inferior thyroid artery (a branch of the thyrocervical trunk of the first part of the subclavian artery) and rarely the small thyroidea ima, which arises from the aorta to supply the isthmus. Venous drainage is through the superior and middle thyroid veins to the internal jugular veins and via the inferior thyroid veins to the brachiocephalic veins (usually on the left). The arterial supply and venous drainage are important to know about when considering thyroid surgery.

The thyroid gland is stimulated by TSH (which is produced from the anterior lobe of the pituitary gland) to produce tri-iodothyronine or T_3 and thyroxine or T_4 – hormones that play an important role in basal metabolic rate.

14   D   The genioglossus muscle causes the tongue to protrude

The tongue is composed of striated, voluntary or skeletal muscle, not smooth muscle. The tongue assists in the formation of a food bolus and propagation towards the back of the mouth and thence into the oesophagus. It also plays a key role in the suckling reflex in neonates, in the articulation of speech and the special sense of taste. Its epithelium is composed of stratified squamous (protective) epithelium because, similar to the skin, it is subject to 'wear and tear'. Tumours arising from the tongue are therefore typically squamous cell carcinomas.

Special taste sensation is by way of the chorda tympani division of the facial nerve for the anterior two-thirds of the tongue and the glossopharyngeal nerve for the posterior third of the tongue. Taste sensation on the anterior two-thirds of the tongue is therefore commonly lost in a facial nerve (or Bell's) palsy. Somatic sensation is by way of the mandibular division of the trigeminal nerve for the anterior two-thirds of the tongue (lingual nerve) and the glossopharyngeal nerve for the posterior third of the tongue.

All the muscles of the tongue are supplied by the hypoglossal nerve, or cranial nerve XII, with the exception of the palatoglossus muscle, which is supplied by the pharyngeal plexus of nerves (IX, X and sympathetics). The hypoglossal nerve may be injured in a carotid endarterectomy or submandibular gland procedures. The most important muscle to know about is the genioglossus muscle, which causes protrusion of the tongue. When genioglossal muscle tone is lost, as in someone with a decreased level of consciousness or a fractured mandible (where the genioglossus muscle arises), the tongue falls back and obstructs the airway, rapidly resulting in hypoxia and death if basic life support measures are not quickly instigated.

15 ▶ D   Are all supplied by the inferior thyroid artery

The parathyroid glands are pinkish/brown glands usually found on the posterior aspect of the thyroid gland. They are usually four in number, two on each side (in 90% of individuals), but can vary from two to six. Each weighs about 50 mg and measures 6 × 3 × 2 mm. The superior parathyroid glands arise from the fourth branchial pouch, whereas the inferior parathyroids are third branchial pouch derivatives. The thymus gland also derives, however, from the third branchial pouch, so the inferior parathyroid glands may get dragged down with the thymus into the mediastinum, making the position of the inferior parathyroid glands highly variable. The superior glands are more constant in position.

The parathyroid glands are all usually supplied by the inferior thyroid artery. A consequence of this is that this artery should always be preserved during a total thyroidectomy to prevent ischaemia of the parathyroid glands, which would render the patient hypocalcaemic and mean that the patient would have to take calcium supplements lifelong.

The parathyroid glands secrete parathyroid hormone (PTH) from chief (or principal) cells. PTH plays an essential role in calcium homoeostasis. However, calcitonin is secreted by the parafollicular cells of the thyroid gland. A parathyroid adenoma is a benign tumour usually of one (but sometimes more) parathyroid gland, which leads to the overproduction of PTH and hypercalcaemia. Treatment consists of neck exploration and removal of the problematic parathyroid adenoma (parathyroidectomy). Care must be taken to avoid damaging the recurrent laryngeal nerves. Exposure of the thymus through a median sternotomy may rarely be necessary, given the liability of the inferior parathyroid glands to end up in unusual positions.

16 ▶ D Lateral rectus is supplied by the abducens nerve

The extraocular muscles are innervated by the third (oculomotor), fourth (trochlear) and sixth (abducens) cranial nerves. The trochlear nerve supplies only one muscle – the superior oblique. The abducens nerve also supplies only one muscle – the lateral rectus. This may be remembered by SO4, LR6. All the remaining muscles are supplied by the oculomotor nerve, ie superior rectus, inferior rectus, inferior oblique and medial rectus are all supplied by the oculomotor, or third, cranial nerve. Injury to any of these cranial nerves (III, IV or VI) may result in ophthalmoplegia and double vision (diplopia).

The recti muscles are easily understood because they move the eyeball in the respective directions indicated by their name. The superior and inferior obliques are more difficult to understand. The superior oblique muscle moves the cornea downwards and outwards, whereas the inferior oblique muscle moves it upwards and inwards. The reason for this is that the oblique muscles pass posteriorly to attach behind the axis of movement, therefore imparting movement opposite to their suggested names. Weakness of the extraocular muscles may occur in the autoimmune condition myasthenia gravis.

Levator palpebrae superioris is the exception to the above. It elevates the eyelid but has a dual innervation from both the oculomotor nerve and sympathetic fibres. The latter innervate a small smooth muscle portion of the levator muscle known as Müller's muscle. The clinical significance of this dual innervation is that a third cranial nerve (oculomotor) palsy, or sympathetic interruption (Horner's syndrome), may result in a droopy eyelid (ptosis). To distinguish the two, it is essential to lift up the eyelid and inspect the pupil to see if it is enlarged (mydriasis in oculomotor nerve palsy) or constricted (miosis in Horner's syndrome). Furthermore, in an oculomotor palsy the eyeball points downwards and outwards from the unopposed action of superior oblique and lateral rectus, supplied by cranial nerves IV and VI. Horner's syndrome is associated with hemifacial anhidrosis (lack of sweating of the ipsilateral face), flushing symptoms (so-called Harlequin syndrome) and enophthalmos (a sunken eyeball), in addition to ptosis and miosis.

17   D   May cause referred pain to the ear if inflamed

The palatine tonsils ('tonsils') are a large collection of lymphoid tissue that project into the oropharynx from the tonsillar fossa, between the palatoglossal arch (in front) and the palatopharyngeal arch (behind). They are most prominent in early life and regress in later years as the lymphoid tissue atrophies. The surface marking is medial to the lower masseter. The palatine, lingual, pharyngeal ('adenoids') and tubal tonsils collectively form an interrupted circle of protective lymphoid tissue at the upper end of the respiratory and alimentary tracts known as Waldeyer's ring. This area has a role in priming lymphocytes for antigens during the early years of life.

The floor of the tonsillar fossa (lateral wall) is the lower part of the superior constrictor, with styloglossus on its lateral side. The luminal surface of the tonsil is covered by non-keratinised, stratified, squamous epithelium, which deeply invaginates the tonsil, forming blind-ended tonsillar crypts. The tonsillar branch of the facial artery (in turn a branch of the external carotid artery) forms the main arterial supply. It enters the tonsil by piercing the superior constrictor.

The main function of the tonsils is immunological, especially in the early years of life. As they harbour microbes, this makes them vulnerable to infection and inflammation (tonsillitis). Lymphatics channels pierce the superior constrictor to reach the deep cervical nodes, especially the jugulodigastric (or tonsillar) node below the angle of the mandible. This is the lymph node that is most commonly enlarged in tonsillitis (jugulodigastric lymphadenopathy).

The mucous membrane overlying the tonsil is supplied mainly by the tonsillar branch of the glossopharyngeal nerve. The glossopharyngeal nerve also supplies the middle ear through its tympanic branch, which explains why tonsillitis commonly causes referred pain to the middle ear. Ear pain may also feature in the early postoperative period after tonsillectomy.

Tonsillectomy (removal of the tonsils) is indicated for recurrent episodes of tonsillitis or obstructive sleep apnoea. Removal does not appear to compromise immune function. The main complication after tonsillectomy is haemorrhage and the usual cause is venous, rather than arterial, bleeding from the external palatine, or paratonsillar, vein. The close proximity of the internal carotid artery (which lies 2.5 cm posterolateral) to the palatine tonsil must be borne in mind at tonsillectomy in order to prevent inadvertent injury.

C Trapezius

The spinal accessory nerve is a branch of cranial nerve XI. It has been given the name spinal accessory because it originates from the upper end of the spinal cord (spinal roots C1–5). It passes through the foramen magnum and 'hitches a ride' with the cranial accessory nerve originating in the nucleus ambiguus. It passes out of the skull by way of the jugular foramen. Its function is to supply only two muscles in the neck – the sternocleidomastoid and trapezius muscles.

Stylopharyngeus is innervated by the glossopharyngeal nerve and palatoglossus is supplied by the pharyngeal plexus (IX, X and sympathetics). Buccinator, on the other hand, is regarded as a muscle of facial expression and is therefore innervated by the facial nerve. Consequently, in facial nerve (Bell's) palsy, food may collect in the vestibule of the mouth.

The surface marking of the spinal accessory nerve is important. It traverses the posterior triangle of the neck from a third of the way down the posterior border of sternocleidomastoid to a third of the way up the anterior border of trapezius, where it terminates ('rule of thirds'). It is vulnerable to iatrogenic injury in procedures that necessitate dissection within the posterior triangle of the neck, such as excision biopsy of a lymph node. In a radical en bloc lymph node dissection of the neck for malignant disease, the spinal accessory nerve may have to be deliberately sacrificed in order to obtain satisfactory clearance.

Damage to the spinal accessory nerve in the posterior triangle of the neck leads to a predictive weakness of trapezius. This results in an inability to shrug the shoulder on the side where the spinal accessory nerve is affected. The sternocleidomastoid muscle is typically spared because the branch to sternocleidomastoid is given off before the spinal accessory nerve enters the posterior triangle of the neck. Trapezius also plays a role in hyperabduction of the arm, so activities such as combing the hair would become more difficult. In the long term, a trapezius palsy (with dropping of the shoulder) may result in a chronic, disabling neuralgia. This may occur as a result of pain from neurological denervation, adhesive capsulitis of the shoulder joint, traction radiculitis of the brachial plexus or more commonly fatigue.

 19   **C**   Has secretomotor action via the glossopharyngeal and auriculotemporal nerves

The parotid gland is the largest of the major salivary glands. It is mainly a serous gland, with only a few scattered mucinous acini. This explains partly why salivary stones (calculi) are rarely encountered in the parotid gland and found more often in the submandibular gland, where secretions are more mucinous and the gland lies below the opening of the duct (which impedes drainage and encourages stasis).

Anteriorly, the gland overlaps the masseter muscle. The parotid duct (of Stensen), not to be confused with Wharton's duct (which is the submandibular duct), passes forward over the masseter muscle and turns around its anterior border to pierce the buccinator (not the masseter) muscle. The buccinator muscle acts like a sphincter at this point and plays an extremely important role in preventing the reflux of air into the parotid (and hence insufflation) when the intraoral pressure is raised, as when playing a trumpet. The duct opens on the mucous membrane of the cheek opposite the second upper molar tooth.

The parotid gland consists of two lobes: superficial and deep – hence the importance of looking in the mouth in cases where a parotid swelling is present, to look for, or exclude, involvement of the deep lobe. There is no middle lobe, although there may

ANSWERS

MCQs in Applied Basic Sciences for Medical Students: Volume 1

be an accessory lobe. The parotid is surrounded by a tough fascial capsule, derived from the investing layer of deep cervical fascia, which is richly innervated. It is the acute swelling of this fibrous envelope that produces the pain of mumps parotitis, a virus infection of the gland.

From superficial to the deep within the parotid lie the following:

- five terminal branches of the facial nerve (also known as the pes anserinus, or 'goose's foot')
- retromandibular vein
- external carotid artery.

The branches of the facial nerve lie most superficially within the parotid gland and hence are extremely vulnerable to damage in parotid surgery. Thus, if the retromandibular vein comes into view, it is too late – the facial nerve has already been severed! It is important to identify and protect the various branches of the facial nerve, which may be remembered by the mnemonic 'Ten Zulus Baited My Cat':

Ten = **t**emporal branch

Zulus = **z**ygomatic branch

Baited = **b**uccal branch

My = **m**arginal mandibular branch

Cat = **c**ervical branch.

The branches of the facial nerve are also likely to be injured by a malignant tumour of the parotid, which is usually highly invasive and quickly involves the facial nerve, causing a facial paralysis.

The secretomotor supply to the parotid (for secretion of saliva) is by way of parasympathetic fibres of the glossopharyngeal nerve, synapsing in the otic ganglion and relaying onwards to the parotid gland through the auriculotemporal nerve. The importance of knowing this lies in a phenomenon called Frey syndrome, which may occur, not infrequently, after parotid surgery or penetrating trauma to the parotid gland. It is caused by misdirected reinnervation of the auriculotemporal nerve fibres to the sweat glands in the facial skin after injury. The patient may complain of gustatory sweating (ie a stimulus intended for saliva production produces sweating instead).

20   C Contains the pituitary and sphenoidal sinus within its medial wall

The cavernous sinus is one of those tricky areas that is difficult to get your head around. It consists of a plexus of veins that lies alongside the sphenoid in the middle cranial fossa. Blood can flow in either direction in the cavernous sinus, depending on local venous pressures. In addition, there are no valves in the cavernous sinus or its connected veins.

The function of the cavernous sinus is unclear. However, as it surrounds the internal carotid artery, which forms the main blood supply to the brain, some have suggested that the cavernous sinus may have evolved to act as a cooling system for the brain. A sort of counter-current mechanism is set up whereby the venous blood contained within the cavernous sinus may actually draw out heat from the internal carotid artery at its centre, although rupture of the internal carotid artery within the cavernous sinus (usually a result of an internal carotid artery aneurysm, or after trauma) may result in a caroticocavernous fistula.

The walls of the cavernous sinus may be summarised as follows:

- Roof: anterior and posterior clinoid processes with uncus of temporal lobe and internal carotid artery on it, and cranial nerves III and IV into it.

- Floor: greater wing of sphenoid.

- Anterior wall (narrow): medial end of superior orbital fissure, ophthalmic veins, orbit.

- Posterior wall (narrow): dura of posterior fossa, superior and inferior petrosal sinuses, peduncle of brain.

- Medial wall: dura over sphenoid, sella turcica, pituitary, sphenoidal air sinus.

- Lateral wall: dura, temporal lobe, cranial nerves III, IV, Va, Vb in wall (from top to bottom).

- Contents: internal carotid artery (with its associated sympathetic plexus), cranial nerve VI, blood.

Note that the optic nerve is not contained within the cavernous sinus.

The area of facial skin bounded by the upper lip, nose, medial part of cheek and eye is a potentially dangerous area to have an infection (the so-called 'danger area of the face'). An infection in this area may result in thrombosis of the facial vein, with spread of organisms through the inferior ophthalmic vein to the cavernous sinus. This may result in a cavernous sinus thrombosis. Via the superficial middle cerebral vein, such thrombosis may spread to the cerebral hemisphere, which may be fatal unless adequately treated with antibiotics.

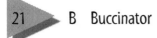

21 B Buccinator

There are four muscles of mastication:

1. Temporalis

2. Masseter

3. Medial pterygoid

4. Lateral pterygoid.

They are all first branchial arch derivatives and therefore innervated by the same nerve (mandibular division of trigeminal, or Vc).

The buccinator muscle is regarded as a muscle of facial expression and is therefore a second branchial arch derivative innervated by the facial, or seventh cranial nerve. This is one of many situations in which a good knowledge of embryology, and especially of the branchial arches, may help to predict the anatomy.

22 ▶ B The anterior communicating artery joins the two anterior cerebral arteries

The internal carotid and vertebral systems anastomose with each other around the optic chiasma and infundibulum of the pituitary stalk at the base of the brain, forming the arterial circle of Willis.

The circle is formed in the following way:

- Posteriorly:

  – at the lower border of the pons, two vertebral arteries combine to form the basilar artery

  – at the upper border of the pons, the basilar artery terminates as right and left posterior cerebral arteries.

- Anteriorly:

  – each internal carotid artery gives off an anterior and middle cerebral artery

  – the circle is completed anteriorly by the single, anterior communicating artery, which connects the two anterior cerebral arteries

  – the circle is completed posteriorly by the two posterior communicating arteries, which connect the posterior cerebral arteries with the internal carotid arteries.

The communicating vessels allow equalisation of blood flow between the two sides of the brain and can allow anastomotic compensation if parts are occluded. However, compensation is not always effective, because of the small size of the blood vessels, and a stroke (or cerebrovascular accident) may result.

Congenital berry aneurysms are abnormal dilatations of blood vessels, usually located around the circle of Willis (because here the tunica media is weakest). Rupture of an aneurysm of the arterial circle accounts for 90% of subarachnoid haemorrhages.

23 ▸ **C A subdural haematoma lies in the plane between the dura mater and the arachnoid mater**

The pia mater is to brain as periosteum is to bone. It is therefore the innermost layer of the meninges and invests the central nervous system to the depths of the deepest fissures and sulci.

The dura mater is the outermost layer of the meninges closest to the bone. It consists of two layers – an outer endosteal layer and inner meningeal layer. The two layers separate to enclose the venous sinuses; folds of the inner layer project into the cranial cavity and are responsible for the formation of the four fibrous flanges, or septa, that minimise rotatory displacement of the brain (falx cerebri, falx cerebelli, tentorium cerebelli and diaphragma sellae). The dura mater is richly innervated and therefore dural stretch causes pain that is commonly experienced as a headache. Two good examples are the headache of meningitis, which is caused by inflammation of the meninges, and a post-lumbar puncture headache, where a headache results from the stimulation of sensory nerve endings in the dura after removal of cerebrospinal fluid (CSF).

The arachnoid mater is a delicate membrane that sits between the dura mater and the pia mater. It is connected to the pia mater by many fine filamentous processes (hence the name arachnoid, or spider-like). The region between the pia mater and the arachnoid mater is the subarachnoid space, filled with CSF. The term 'leptomeninges' refers to the arachnoid and pia maters.

A good understanding of the various meningeal layers is necessary in order to understand the various types of intracranial haemorrhage that may occur.

An extradural haematoma occurs between the endosteal layer of the dura mater and the skull. It is commonly the result of trauma with bleeding from the middle meningeal artery, and is often associated with an underlying fracture (commonly in the region of the pterion, which is the surface marking for the anterior branch of the middle meningeal artery that is commonly implicated). Containment of the arterial bleed may lead to a lucid interval until the pressure builds up to such a point that compression of the brain occurs with resulting coma.

A subdural haematoma is often a result of venous bleeding in the space between the dura mater and the arachnoid mater. It commonly occurs in elderly or demented people, or in people with alcohol problems where shrinkage of the brain occurs. This stretches the bridging veins that run across the surface the brain and makes them vulnerable to tearing. As the bleed is venous rather than arterial, lower pressures result in a more gradual accumulation of blood than an arterial bleed. The result is a gradual deterioration in cognitive function and patients often present with confusion (chronic subdural haematoma).

A subarachnoid haematoma is an arterial bleed that occurs in the subarachnoid space, between the pia and arachnoid. This usually follows rupture of a berry aneurysm in the region of the circle of Willis, which causes blood to contaminate the CSF – visible at lumbar puncture.

Finally, an intracerebral bleed occurs within the brain parenchyma itself and is therefore unrelated to the cranial meninges.

The facial, or seventh, cranial nerve has a variety of different functions and is important clinically. Its functions may be summarised as follows:

- associated developmentally with the second branchial arch
- supplies the muscles of facial expression
- special taste sensation to the anterior two-thirds of the tongue via the chorda tympani nerve
- carries secretomotor fibres to the lacrimal gland through the greater petrosal nerve
- secretomotor to the submandibular and sublingual glands
- somatic sensation to the external auditory meatus.

Special taste from the posterior third of the tongue is carried by the glossopharyngeal nerve. Levator palpebrae superioris, responsible for elevating the eyelid, is not a muscle of facial expression; it is innervated by the oculomotor nerve and sympathetics. Orbicularis oculi, responsible for blinking and screwing the eye tight, is regarded as a muscle of facial expression and is supplied by the facial nerve.

The four principal muscles of mastication (temporalis, medial and lateral pterygoids, masseter) are all supplied by the mandibular division of the trigeminal nerve. Note that buccinator is not a muscle of mastication and is innervated by the facial nerve.

Understanding of the above helps to explain what happens when things go wrong. A facial nerve (Bell's) palsy results in weakness of the muscles of facial expression down one side of the face, leading to a droopy face. Note that this is a lower motor neuron palsy and that all the muscles down the side of the face are affected, including the forehead muscles. This is in sharp contrast to a cerebrovascular accident, or upper motor neuron facial palsy, where the upper (forehead) muscles are spared because they are bilaterally innervated from both cerebral cortices.

Apart from a droopy face, however, a Bell's palsy also results in loss of sensation to the anterior two-thirds of the tongue and hyperacusis (sensitivity to sounds), as a result of dennervation of the stapedius muscle, which normally serves to dampen down sounds in the middle ear. Dry eyes occur as a result of the loss of the secretomotor supply to the lacrimal gland (and hence the need to protect the eye to prevent keratitis and corneal ulceration in a facial nerve palsy). This is exacerbated by denervation of orbicularis oculi, which normally functions to spread the tear film over the surface of the cornea with the blinking reflex.

Although it may not seem very important, the small somatic sensory branch of the facial nerve (which supplies the external auditory meatus) may explain why, in Ramsay Hunt syndrome (herpes zoster infection of the geniculate ganglion), herpes vesicles are found around the external auditory meatus,

This question illustrates quite nicely how a good understanding of anatomy may help the student in future clinical practice.

25 ▶ B The invertebral joints are secondary cartilaginous joints

The spinal cord terminates at L1–2. Below this only nerve roots exist within the vertebral canal (cauda equina). It is therefore safe to perform a lumbar puncture at the L3–4 or L4–5 level. Fortunately, for the purpose of a lumbar puncture, the dural sac containing the CSF does not terminate until S2.

The intervertebral joints are secondary cartilaginous joints. Between each vertebral body lies an intervertebral disc that is predominantly created from an annulus fibrosus of fibrocartilage with an internal nucleus pulposus, a bubble of semiliquid gelatinous substance derived from the embryonic notochord. With age the fibrocartilaginous annulus does deteriorate and may weaken, often in the lower lumbar region, giving rise to a slipped, or prolapsed, disc. In such cases the nucleus pulposus is typically extruded posterolaterally.

The relationship of the nerve roots to intervertebral discs is of great importance. At the L4–5 level, the fourth lumbar nerve roots within their dural sheath have already emerged from the intervertebral foramen and so are not lying low enough to come into contact with the disc. The roots that lie behind the posterolateral part of this disc are those of the fifth lumbar nerve, which are the ones likely to be irritated by the prolapse. Thus, the general rule throughout the vertebral column is that, when a disc herniates (usually posterolaterally, rather than in the midline), it may irritate the nerve roots that are one below the disc.

The spinal cord is supplied by the single anterior spinal artery and two (right and left) posterior spinal arteries. As there is only one anterior spinal artery, the spinal cord is vulnerable to anterior ischaemia (the anterior spinal artery syndrome). The posterior columns (mediating light touch and proprioception) remain intact, but most of the rest of the cord below the level of the lesion is affected, leading to weakness (corticospinal tract involvement) and loss of pain/temperature sensation (anterolateral, or spinothalamic, tract involvement).

The richly supplied red marrow of the vertebral body drains through its posterior surface via large basivertebral veins into Batson's internal vertebral venous plexus, which lies inside the vertebral canal but outside the dura (in the extradural space). It drains into the external vertebral venous plexus and thence into regional segmental veins. These veins are valveless and often act as a subsidiary route for blood flow when the inferior vena cava cannot cope, with a sudden flush of blood resulting from a sudden increase of intra-abdominal pressure (eg straining, coughing, sneezing). A rise in pressure on the abdominal and pelvic veins would tend to force the blood backward out of the abdominal and pelvic cavities into the valveless veins within the vertebral canal. The existence of this venous plexus may explain how carcinoma of the prostate, kidney, breast, bronchus and thyroid may metastasise to the vertebral column.

Thorax
Answers

26   ▶   **D**   Has lymphatics that have connections with those of the opposite breasts

The base of the breast is fairly constant, from the sternal edge to the midaxillary line and from the second to the sixth rib. Two-thirds of its base overlies pectoralis major and a third overlaps onto serratus anterior. Contraction of the underlying pectoralis major muscle (a woman puts her hands on her hips and pushes in) exacerbates any asymmetry between the breasts (eg as a result of a breast cancer) and is a clinically useful manoeuvre.

The breast's main purpose is lactation. The organ enlarges in pregnancy in preparation for lactation. After the menopause, involution (atrophy) occurs, hence mammograms are less useful in young women (when the breast tissue is dense and cancers do not show up as well), although they are more useful at the time of the menopause and beyond, when breast tissue is composed mainly of fat (less dense on mammography), enabling cancers to show up more clearly.

The blood supply to the breast is mainly derived from the lateral thoracic artery (a branch of the second part of the axillary artery). However, the internal thoracic, thoracoacromial and posterior intercostal arteries also send branches to the breast.

The lymph drainage is of considerable anatomical and clinical importance because of the frequent development of cancer in the gland and the subsequent dissemination of malignant cells along the lymphatics to the lymph nodes. Around 75% of the lymphatic drainage of the breast passes to 20–30 or so axillary lymph nodes. They are usually described as lying in the following groups, which can be remembered by the mnemonic, APICAL:

A = **a**nterior (or pectoral) group

P = **p**osterior (or subscapular) group

I = **i**nfraclavicular (or deltopectoral) group

C = **c**entral group

A = **a**pical group

L = **l**ateral (or brachial) group.

The medial quadrants of the breast (where fortunately cancer is less common) enter the thorax to drain into the internal mammary lymph nodes alongside the internal thoracic artery. Thoracic lymph nodes are difficult, or impossible, to treat, but the lymph nodes of the axilla can be removed surgically.

The superficial lymphatics of the breast have connections with those of the opposite breast, anterior abdominal wall and supraclavicular lymph nodes. These tend to convey lymph from the breast when the other channels are obstructed by malignant disease, or after their destruction by radiotherapy or surgery.

B The direction of fibres of the external intercostal muscle is downwards and medial

The intercostal neurovascular bundle lies in a groove on the undersurface of each rib, running in the plane between the internal and innermost intercostal muscles.

The vein, artery and nerve lie in that order, from above downwards, under cover of the lower border of the rib. This may be remembered by VAN:

V = **v**ein

A = **a**rtery

N = **n**erve.

Thus, a needle or trocar for drainage, or aspiration, of fluid from the pleural cavity is inserted just above the rib in order to avoid the main vessels and nerves.

The fibres of the external intercostals muscle pass obliquely downwards and forwards from the sharp lower border of the rib above to the smooth upper border of the rib below. This may be remembered because it follows the same direction as having one's hands in one's pockets. Although important for the mechanics of respiration, the diaphragm is the main muscle of respiration.

ANSWERS

28   D   It lacks a true serosal surface

The oesophagus is a segmental muscular tube running from the cricoid ring, at the level of C6, to the cardia of the stomach. It is 25 cm long (with the distance from the upper incisor teeth to the lower oesophageal sphincter being approximately 40 cm). These distances are useful to learn for the purposes of endoscopy. The upper third of the oesophagus consists of skeletal muscle (voluntary muscle that initiates swallowing), but then there is a progressive change to smooth muscle, such that the lower third of the oesophagus consists of only smooth muscle.

The blood supply and lymphatic drainage are segmental. The upper third of the oesophagus is supplied by the inferior thyroid artery and the lymphatics drain to the deep cervical group of lymph nodes. The middle third of the oesophagus is supplied directly by branches from the descending thoracic aorta, and the lymphatics drain to the preaortic and para-aortic lymph nodes. The lower third of the oesophagus is supplied by the left gastric artery, and the lymphatics drain to the coeliac group of lymph nodes. However, within the oesophageal walls there are lymphatic channels that enable lymph to pass for long distances within the viscus, so that drainage from any given area does not strictly follow the above pattern.

The surface epithelium is largely non-keratinising, stratified, squamous epithelium. This is normally replaced by columnar epithelium at the gastro-oesophageal junction, but columnar epithelium may line the lower oesophagus. An oesophagus that has the squamocolumnar junction 3 cm or more above the gastro-oesophageal junction is abnormal and called Barrett's oesophagus. This is a metaplastic change that takes place in response to acid reflux and is a premalignant condition.

Except for the short intra-abdominal segment of the oesophagus there is no serosal surface. This is important to know about for two reasons: first, it makes the oesophagus vulnerable to anastomotic leakage in the postoperative period; second, as the oesophagus lacks a serosal covering, oesophageal carcinoma encounters few anatomical barriers to local invasion.

29 ▶ C The narrowest part of the oesophagus is at the level of cricopharyngeus

There are four classic points along the oesophagus where constrictions take place.

1. Cricopharyngeus sphincter, 15 cm from the incisor teeth, which is the narrowest part of the oesophagus. Its function is to prevent air entering the oesophagus and stomach. The cricopharyngeus sphincter relaxes with the swallowing reflex.

2. Where the oesophagus is crossed by the aortic arch, 22 cm from the incisor teeth.

3. Where the oesophagus is crossed by the left principal bronchus, 27 cm from the incisor teeth.

4. Where the oesophagus passes through the opening in the diaphragm, 38 cm from the incisor teeth.

Although the left atrium is in front of the lower part of the oesophagus below the left bronchus, it is only when enlarged (eg in mitral valve disease) that the left atrium causes an indentation in the oesophagus, resulting in difficulty swallowing or dysphagia.

These constrictions are of considerable clinical importance because they are sites where swallowed foreign bodies can lodge, or through which it may be difficult to pass an oesophagoscope. As a slight delay in the passage of food or fluid occurs at these levels, strictures commonly develop here after drinking caustic fluids. These constrictions are also common sites of carcinoma of the oesophagus.

The lower oesophageal sphincter is not a true anatomical sphincter, but a functional one. Maintenance of the lower oesophageal sphincter is largely brought about through the following features:

- the effect of the right crus of the diaphragm forming a 'sling' around the lower oesophagus

- the oblique angle that the oesophagus takes on entering the gastric cardia (angle of His), acting as a flap–valve mechanism

- greater intra-abdominal than intragastric pressure acting to compress the abdominal part of the oesophagus

- mucosal rosette (prominent folds at the gastro-oesophageal junction)

- phrenico-oesophageal ligament (fold of connective tissue)

- the effect of gastrin in increasing lower oesophageal sphincter tone

- unidirectional peristalsis.

A problematic lower oesophageal sphincter may lead to problems, such as gastro-oesophageal reflux disease, hiatus hernia or a condition known as achalasia.

C Forms the main muscle of respiration at rest

The diaphragm is a musculotendinous structure composed of outer skeletal muscle fibres and a central tendinous region. It partitions the thoracic cavity from the abdominal cavity and is the main muscle of respiration at rest (accounting for 70% of inspiration at rest). On inspiration, the diaphragm contracts, which lowers the diaphragm. This decreases pressure within the thoracic cavity and air moves into the lungs, resulting in lung inflation. On expiration, the diaphragm relaxes and the diaphragm moves up.

The diaphragm receives motor innervation from the phrenic nerve (C3, C4, C5). (C3, C4, C5, keep the diaphragm alive!) The diaphragm has no other motor supply besides the phrenic nerve, which is why cervical spine injuries with injury to the cervical spinal cord can be so disastrous, and hence the importance of proper cervical spine immobilisation in trauma victims.

The phrenic nerve is two-thirds motor and a third sensory. The sensory nerve supply to the diaphragmatic parietal pleura and diaphragmatic peritoneum covering the central surfaces of the diaphragm is from the phrenic nerve. The sensory supply to the periphery of the diaphragm is from the lower six intercostal nerves.

ANSWERS

31

> E   The sympathetic trunks pass posterior to the medial arcuate ligament

A common question!

Vena cava opening (T8):
  inferior vena cava
  right phrenic nerve

Oesophageal opening (T10):
  oesophagus
  left and right vagus nerves (RIP = right is posterior)
  oesophageal branches of left gastric vessels
  lymphatics from lower third of oesophagus

Aortic opening (T12):
  aorta
  azygous and hemiazygous veins
  thoracic duct

Crura (T12):
  greater, lesser and least splanchnic nerves

Behind medial arcuate ligament:
  sympathetic trunks

Behind lateral arcuate ligament:
  subcostal (T12) neurovascular bundle

The left phrenic nerve pierces the muscle of the left dome of the diaphragm.

The inferior vena cava passes through the central tendinous portion of the diaphragm and not the muscular portion of the diaphragm at the level of T8. The reason for this is clear – if the vena cava passed through the muscular part of the diaphragm, each time the diaphragm contracted with respiration it would obstruct venous return, causing syncope.

C   Crosses the midline at the level of T5

The thoracic duct is 45 cm long and starts at T12 from the cisterna chyli, which lies to the right of the aorta. It drains all the lymph below the diaphragm, left thorax, and left head and neck regions. Valves are present along the duct and encourage the propagation of chyle along the duct.

The duct ascends behind the right crus and to the right of the aorta and oesophagus. It crosses the midline to the left, posterior to the oesophagus, at the level of T5. It passes over the dome of the left pleura, anterior to the left vertebral and subclavian arteries, and enters the confluence of the left subclavian and internal jugular veins.

The equivalent of the thoracic duct on the right is the right lymphatic trunk. This drains on the right into the confluence of the right subclavian and internal jugular veins.

Injury to the thoracic duct may occur after trauma or during insertion of a central venous catheter on the left-hand side. This can result in a chylothorax (a collection of lymph within the thoracic cavity). A haemothorax is a collection of blood.

33 ▶ E The lungs receive a dual blood supply

The right and left lungs are not mirror images of each other. Although the right lung is made up of three lobes, the left lung possesses only two lobes. Each of the lobes, in turn, is separated by fissures or interlobar clefts. Thus, on the right, there must be two fissures separating three separate lobes (the oblique and horizontal fissures, respectively). On the left, there is only one fissure separating the two lobes – the oblique fissure. Thus, the horizontal fissure exists only on the right.

There are typically 10 anatomically definable bronchopulmonary segments within each lung, each containing a segmental (tertiary) bronchus, a segmental artery, a segmental vein, lymphatics and autonomic nerves, and separated from their adjacent segments by connective tissue. Each is pyramidal in shape with its apex towards the lung root and its base towards the surface of the lung, and each is anatomically and functionally separate from the rest. The importance of understanding bronchopulmonary segments is that diseased segments, as they are structural units, can be selectively removed surgically (segmentectomy). Nowadays this can be performed by video-assisted thoracoscopic surgery (VATS).

The right bronchus is shorter, wider and more vertical than the left bronchus, so that foreign bodies that fall down the trachea are more likely to enter the right bronchus. Furthermore, material aspirated by a supine, comatose or anaesthetised patient would tend to gravitate into the apical segment of the right lower lobe, which is consequently a common site for aspiration pneumonia and abscess formation.

The lungs receive a dual blood supply by way of the pulmonary artery and the bronchial arteries. Thus, obstruction of a small pulmonary arteriole by a pulmonary embolus has no effect in an otherwise healthy individual with an intact bronchial circulation.

In such circumstances, pulmonary embolism usually results only in infarction when the circulation is already inadequate, as in patients with heart or lung disease. A large embolus that impacts in the main pulmonary artery, or lodges at the bifurcation (as a saddle embolus would), results in sudden death.

34 ▶ B It extends above the clavicle superiorly

The pleura clothes each lung and lines the thoracic cavity. It is composed of two layers. The visceral layer on the lung surface is in contact with the parietal pleura, which lines the thoracic wall (rib cage, vertebra, diaphragm), the surfaces being lubricated by a thin film of fluid. The space in between the two layers is known as the pleural space or cavity.

The parietal pleura (along with the apex of the lung) projects 2.5 cm above the medial third of the clavicle superiorly. A penetrating wound above the medial end of the clavicle may therefore involve the apex of the lung, resulting in a pneumothorax (collapsed lung). This is most commonly seen as an iatrogenic complication during the insertion of a subclavian (central) venous line. As a result of the obliquity of the thoracic inlet, the pleura does not extend above the neck of the first rib, which lies well above the clavicle.

It is also important to remember that the lower limit of the pleural reflection, as seen from the back, lies below the medial border of the twelfth rib, behind the upper border of the kidney. It is vulnerable to damage here during removal of the kidney (nephrectomy) through an incision in the loin. Proper identification of the twelfth rib is essential to avoid entering the pleural cavity.

The visceral pleura is poorly innervated, has an autonomic nerve supply and is insensitive to ordinary stimuli. The parietal pleura, on the other hand, receives a rich innervation from the intercostal nerves and the phrenic nerve, and is sensitive to pain. Thus, in tuberculosis or pneumonia pain may never be experienced. However, once lung disease crosses the visceral pleura to involve the parietal pleura, pain becomes a prominent feature. Lobar pneumonia with pleurisy is a good example. As the lower part of the costal parietal pleura receives its innervation from the lower five intercostal nerves, which also innervate the skin of the lower anterior abdominal wall, pleurisy in this area commonly produces pain that is referred to the abdomen. This has sometimes resulted in a mistaken diagnosis of an acute abdominal lesion. In a similar manner, pleurisy of the central part of the diaphragmatic pleura, which receives sensory innervation from the phrenic nerve (C3, C4, C5), can lead to referred pain over the shoulder, because the skin of this region is supplied by the supraclavicular nerves (C3, C4).

The reflections (and therefore the surface anatomy) of the pleural linings and lungs may be remembered by the '2, 4, 6, 8, 10, 12 rule', ie:

Pleura:

- Starts 2.5 cm above the mid-point of medial third of the clavicle
- Meets in midline at the second rib
- Left side diverges at the fourth rib (to make room for the heart)
- Right side continues parasternally to the sixth rib
- Both cross the eighth rib in the mid-clavicular line
- Both pleurae cross the tenth rib in mid-axillary line
- Both reach posterior chest just below the twelfth rib

Lung:

- Below the sixth rib, the lungs extend to two rib spaces less than the pleura (ie opposite the sixth rib's mid-clavicular line, eighth rib's mid-axillary line and the tenth rib posteriorly). The parietal pleura extends a further two rib spaces more inferiorly than the inferior lung edge, to allow space for lung expansion.

Note how the right and left reflections are not identical to each other. On the left it is displaced by the central position of the heart.

 35   C   It is responsible for the formation of the transverse and oblique sinuses

The pericardium refers to the sac that encloses the heart. It is made up of three layers: an outer fibrous pericardium and an inner serous pericardium (which comprises both an outer parietal layer and an inner visceral layer). A small amount of pericardial fluid exists between the visceral and parietal layers of the serous pericardium. This allows the heart to move freely within the pericardial sac.

The pericardium serves two main functions. First, it protects and lubricates the heart. Second, it contributes to diastolic coupling of the left and right ventricles. However, cardiac contractility functions normally (although possibly not optimally) in the absence of a pericardium. Indeed, after coronary artery bypass grafting surgery, the pericardium is often left open (pericardiotomy) to prevent a tamponade effect caused by the build-up of fluid in the postoperative period.

Between the parietal and visceral layers there are two pericardial sinuses. The transverse sinus lies in between the pulmonary artery and aorta in front and the pulmonary veins and superior vena cava behind. The oblique sinus is a space behind the heart between the left atrium in front and the fibrous pericardium behind, posterior to which lies the oesophagus. The transverse sinus is especially important in cardiac surgery. A digit and ligature can be passed through the transverse sinus and, by tightening the ligature, the surgeon can stop the blood flow through the aorta or pulmonary trunk while cardiac surgery is performed.

The fibrous pericardium and the parietal layer of the serous pericardium receive a rich innervation from the phrenic nerve. However, the visceral layer is insensitive. The pain of pericardial inflammation (pericarditis) is pronounced, originates in the parietal layer and is transmitted by way of the phrenic nerve.

If extensive fluid collects within the pericardial cavity, it interferes with the action of the heart because the fibrous pericardium is inelastic. The pericardial cavity, in this way, behaves like a rigid box with only a finite amount of space. Thus, if the pressure builds up within the compartment, something else has to give and this usually results in compression of the heart. Such a situation is most commonly encountered in the case of penetrating trauma, where the build-up of blood within the pericardial space often results in a cardiac tamponade, manifesting as a precipitous fall in cardiac output. Pericardiocentesis (removal, by needle, of pericardial fluid) may be a life-saving manoeuvre in such circumstances.

D Occlusion of the anterior interventricular artery (left anterior descending artery) results in an anterior myocardial infarction

The heart is composed of cardiac muscle. This cardiac muscle receives the oxygen and nutrients that it requires to pump effectively through the coronary arteries. There are two principal coronary arteries – the right and left coronary arteries.

The right coronary artery originates from the anterior aortic sinus, whereas the left coronary artery originates from the left posterior aortic sinus. The left coronary artery divides into an anterior interventricular (or left anterior descending) artery and circumflex branches. The right coronary artery gives off the posterior interventricular (posterior descending) artery. It supplies the right atrium and part of the left atrium, the SA node in 60% of cases, the right ventricle, the posterior part of the interventricular septum and the AV node in 80% of cases. The left coronary artery supplies the left atrium, left ventricle, anterior interventricular septum, SA node in 40% of cases and AV node in of 20% of cases.

By understanding the above, you can predict the consequences of a blockage within a particular coronary artery. Thus, a lesion within the anterior interventricular artery (of the left coronary artery) leads to an anterior myocardial infarct and death of the left ventricular muscle, resulting in congestive cardiac failure. A lesion within the right coronary artery would be expected to produce arrhythmias because the dominant arterial supply to the SA and AV nodes is through the right coronary artery.

Angina pectoris originates in the muscle or vessels, and is transmitted by sympathetic nerves. The pain of angina is often referred to the left arm and shoulder, but also frequently to the neck, throat and even the side of the face. The reason for this is that the heart originates during embryonic life in the neck, as do the arms. Therefore, both these structures receive pain fibres from the same spinal segments. Angina is usually a result of the laying down of fatty deposits within the coronary arteries (atherosclerosis). However, angina may also occur in the absence of atherosclerosis, in cases such as aortic stenosis, cocaine abuse, vasculitis and variant (Prinzmetal's) angina; the last is caused by vasospasm of the coronary arteries.

Abdomen and pelvis
Answers

 37 ▶ **D** The posterior wall of the canal is bounded by transversalis fascia and the conjoint tendon medially

Many students are troubled by the anatomy and significance of the inguinal canal. The following are its boundaries.

- Anterior wall:
    - skin, superficial fascia, external oblique (for whole length)
    - internal oblique for lateral third.

- Posterior wall:
    - transversalis fascia (for whole length)
    - conjoint tendon and pectineal (Cooper's) ligament medially.

- Floor:
    - inguinal ligament (Poupart's ligament).

- Roof:
    - arching fibres of internal oblique muscle and transversus abdominis, which fuse to form the conjoint tendon on the posteromedial aspect of the canal.

The inguinal canal is an oblique passage that runs from the deep to the superficial inguinal rings and serves to transmit the testis (in the developing male) and spermatic cord in adulthood. It therefore functions to exteriorise the testis, so that an optimal temperature can be obtained in order for spermatogenesis to proceed. In the female, the inguinal canal transmits the round ligament of the uterus, and by this means helps to maintain and support the uterus in its typical anteverted, anteflexed position.

The deep inguinal ring is a hole in the transversalis fascia and lies a finger-breadth above the mid-inguinal point (ie halfway between the anterosuperior iliac spine and pubic tubercle). The superficial inguinal ring is a hole in the external oblique aponeurosis. The key to understanding the inguinal canal is to concentrate on the internal oblique layer that laterally forms the anterior wall of the inguinal canal. The internal oblique then arches over the top of the canal forming its roof and blends with the transversus abdominis layer posteriorly and medially to form the conjoint tendon.

A hernia is simply a protrusion of a viscus, or part of a viscus, outwith its normal position. A femoral hernia can be distinguished from an inguinal hernia by its position. An inguinal hernia lies above and medial to the pubic tubercle, whereas a femoral hernia lies below and lateral to it. The pubic tubercle is thus an important landmark in differentiating a femoral from an inguinal hernia. In addition, an inguinal hernia may be either direct or indirect. A direct hernia passes straight through a weakness in the anterior abdominal wall and through the superficial ring only. An indirect hernia, on the other hand, passes through both the deep and superficial inguinal rings, and thereby passes along the entire length of the inguinal canal.

E The epiploic foramen forms the entrance to the lesser sac

The greater and lesser sacs of the peritoneal cavity communicate with each other by way of the epiploic foramen (of Winslow). This is therefore a key landmark within the abdomen from both an anatomical and a clinical point of view.

The boundaries of the epiploic foramen are as follows:

- Anteriorly: the lesser omentum with the common bile duct, portal vein and common hepatic artery in its free edge.
- Posteriorly: inferior vena cava.
- Superiorly: the caudate (not the quadrate) lobe of the liver.
- Inferiorly: first part of duodenum.
- Medially: lesser sac (posterior to stomach).
- Laterally: greater sac.

From a clinical standpoint, the epiploic foramen is important for two reasons: first, it may be the site of internal herniation of bowel and, second, compression of the common hepatic artery in the free edge of the lesser omentum by a carefully placed hand in the epiploic foramen may be a life-saving manoeuvre at laparotomy to control bleeding from the liver (Pringle's manoeuvre).

39   A Valvulae conniventes

The following distinguish large bowel from small bowel in the cadaver, at laparotomy and on imaging. Large bowel has the following three characteristic features:

1. Haustra (synonymous with sacculations)

2. Appendices epiploicae

3. Taeniae coli.

Valvulae conniventes (synonymous with plica circulares) are a feature of small bowel rather than large bowel.

The gallbladder has three main functions: it stores bile, concentrates bile (5- to 20-fold) and adds mucus to the bile secreted by the liver. It has a capacity of about 50 mL. Its mucous membrane is a lax areolar tissue lined with simple columnar epithelium. Under the epithelium there is a layer of connective tissue, followed by a muscular wall that contracts in response to cholecystokinin, a peptide hormone secreted by the duodenal mucosa in response to the entry of fatty foods into the duodenum.

The gallbladder is supplied by the cystic artery, usually a branch of the right hepatic artery. It runs across the triangle formed by the liver, common hepatic duct and cystic duct to reach the gallbladder (Calot's triangle). Calot's triangle reliably contains the cystic artery, cystic lymph node (of Lund), connective tissue and lymphatics. It is important to dissect out this triangle at laparoscopic cholecystectomy in order to successfully identify and ligate the cystic artery before removal of the gallbladder.

The gallbladder is not essential for life. Indeed rats and horses manage perfectly well without gallbladders. Patients who have had their gallbladders removed lead a normal life and can expect a normal life expectancy. Removal of the gallbladder (cholecystectomy) is a common operation. Indications usually relate to gallstone disease, but rarely it may be performed for conditions such as carcinoma of the gallbladder. It may be performed open, but nowadays is mostly performed by the laparoscopic (keyhole) route.

ANSWERS

Abdomen and pelvis – Answers

41   B   Gallbladder disease may refer pain to the right shoulder tip

The surface marking of the gallbladder is opposite the tip of the right ninth costal cartilage, ie where the lateral edge of the right rectus sheath crosses the costal margin. This is an important landmark because it is the site of maximal abdominal tenderness in gallbladder disease.

Gallstone disease may refer pain to the right shoulder tip (Kehr's sign). There is an important anatomical explanation underlying this phenomenon. An inflamed or distended gallbladder may irritate the diaphragm that is supplied by the phrenic nerve (C3, C4, C5, keeps the diaphragm alive!). These very same nerve roots also provide sensation to the right shoulder tip by way of the supraclavicular nerves (C3, C4, C5). The body misinterprets the signals that it receives and interprets the pain signals as coming from the right shoulder tip. This is the concept of referred pain (pain felt remote from the site of tissue damage). The very same phenomenon may occur in a ruptured ectopic pregnancy, or splenic rupture, but in this instance the diaphragmatic irritant is free blood within the peritoneal cavity. Indeed, anything that irritates the diaphragm may cause referred pain to the right shoulder tip.

Courvoisier's law states that, in the presence of obstructive jaundice, a palpable gallbladder is unlikely to result from gallstones, because gallstones cause chronic inflammation, fibrosis and a shrunken gallbladder. Rather, the law implies that a palpable gallbladder is more likely to result from carcinoma of the head of pancreas causing an obstruction to biliary outflow. Note, however, that the law is not true the other way round (ie in the presence of obstructive jaundice an impalpable gallbladder is always the result of gallstones) because 50% of dilated gallbladders cannot be palpated on clinical examination, as a result of either the patient's obesity or overlap of the liver.

Cholelithiasis (ie the presence of gallstones) is a common condition. Often gallstones are picked up incidentally on ultrasonography. The stones are of two types: calcium bilirubinate and cholesterol stones. In Europe and the USA, 85% of the stones are cholesterol stones. Three factors seem to be involved in the formation of cholesterol stones – bile stasis, supersaturation of bile with cholesterol (lithogenic bile) and nucleation factors. Crucially, however, 80% of patients with gallstones remain asymptomatic throughout their lives. Therefore, in a patient with proven gallstones on ultrasonography, a good history is imperative in order to assess whether or not the patient's symptoms are really the result of the gallstones. If not, the patient is unlikely to benefit from having the gallbladder removed.

42   E   The right subhepatic space or hepatorenal pouch (of Rutherford-Morison) is the most dependent part of the peritoneal cavity

The liver capsule is composed of two adherent layers: a thick fibrous inner layer called Glisson's capsule (note that Gerota's fascia surrounds the kidney) and an outer serous layer that is derived from the peritoneum.

Glisson's capsule covers the entire surface of the liver and the serous layer covers most of the liver surface, excluding the 'bare' area of the liver near the diaphragm, the porta hepatis, and the area where the gallbladder is attached to the liver. So tough is Glisson's capsule that a subcapsular haematoma occurring as a result of liver parenchymal injury may be effectively contained by the capsule. The capsule is richly innervated by autonomic fibres, and capsular stretching as a result, for example, of malignancy may be intensely painful.

The liver receives a dual blood supply – from the hepatic artery and the portal vein. The portal vein provides 75% of the total hepatic blood flow, the hepatic artery 25%. The portal vein contains blood from the gut, rich in products of digestion, but is only about 85% saturated with oxygen. The hepatic artery oxygen concentration, however, is about 99%. Each vessel therefore supplies approximately equal amounts of oxygen to the liver.

The ligamentum venosum is a remnant of the ductus venosus (a channel that shunts blood from the left umbilical vein directly into the inferior vena cava during gestation, thereby bypassing the liver and preserving oxygenated blood for the head and neck region). The ligamentum teres (or round ligament), in the free edge of the falciform ligament, is a remnant of the left umbilical vein.

Within the peritoneal cavity proper, there are various spaces that are potential sites where pus may collect (forming an abscess). The most important spaces to recognise are the right and left subphrenic (subdiaphragmatic) spaces, the pelvis, the right and left paracolic gutters, and the right subhepatic space (also known as the hepatorenal pouch of Rutherford–Morison). When lying supine, the last space is the most dependent part of the peritoneal cavity and hence it is an area where intraperitoneal fluid is likely to accumulate in the form of an abscess (or 'collection'). The left subhepatic space is the lesser sac.

43   B   Feature at the lower end of the oesophagus

Portosystemic anastomoses are important sites in the body at which the portal venous circulation meets the systemic venous circulation. There are five principal sites where this takes place:

1. Lower end of the oesophagus

2. Upper end of the anal canal

3. Periumbilical region of the anterior abdominal wall

4. Bare area of the liver

5. Retroperitoneum.

In liver failure (cirrhosis), fibrosis of the liver takes place with obliteration of the blood vessels within it. The result is that blood from the portal vein is unable to drain through the liver into the inferior vena cava. Consequently, 80% of the portal blood flow is shunted into collateral channels and only 20% reaches the liver. The portosystemic anastomoses open up in liver failure (but not in renal failure) and act as collateral channels, allowing an alternative path for the flow of blood. Nevertheless, the opening up of the collaterals does not decrease the level of pressure within the portal system and portal hypertension ensues. The consequence of this is splenomegaly as a result of portal hypertension. However, the spleen itself is not a site of portosystemic anastomosis.

The most important area to remember as a site of portosystemic anastomosis is the lower end of the oesophagus because of its clinical significance. The veins from the lower third of the oesophagus drain downwards to the left gastric vein (portal system); above this level, oesophageal veins drain into the azygous and hemiazygous systems (systemic system). Subsequently, in portal hypertension, dilatations of the veins

ANSWERS

MCQs in Applied Basic Sciences for Medical Students: Volume 1

within the lower end of the oesophagus may take place, known as oesophageal varices. The same effect also occurs at the other sites of portosystemic anastomosis, although there is one key difference between the lower oesophagus and these other sites, ie oesophageal varices have thin walls and are prone to rupture, as predicted by LaPlace's law. Rupture of oesophageal varices may result in a catastrophic upper gastrointestinal bleed that is often fatal.

Dilatations of veins within the anterior abdominal wall (also a site of portosystemic anastomosis) are known as caput medusae, because of their resemblance to the hair of the Greek mythological character, Medusa. Venous dilatations within the upper end of the anal canal in portal hypertension may lead to the formation of haemorrhoids. However, in practice, they rarely lead to problems and the presence of oesophageal varices are far more significant.

44 **E If removed from a patient leaves him or her at risk of post-splenectomy sepsis**

The spleen, the largest of the lymphoid organs, lies under the diaphragm on the left side of the abdomen. It may be summarised by 1, 3, 5, 7, 9, 11, ie it measures 1 × 3 × 5 inches, weighs 7 oz (200 g) and lies beneath ribs 9 to 1. The spleen lies at the far left margin of the lesser sac below the diaphragm. Thus, if you place your hand in the lesser sac (via the epiploic foramen of Winslow), the spleen is the most laterally placed structure palpable.

Accessory spleen or splenunculi represent congenital ectopic splenic tissue and are found in up to 20% of individuals. One or several may be found, usually along the splenic vessels or in the peritoneal attachments. They are rarely larger than 2 cm in diameter.

Two 'pedicles', the gastrosplenic and lienorenal ligaments, connect the hilum of the spleen to the greater curvature of the stomach and the anterior surface of the left kidney, respectively. The splenic vessels and pancreatic tail lie in the lienorenal ligament. The short gastric and left gastroepiploic vessels run in the gastrosplenic ligament.

The functions of the spleen may be summarised by FISH:

F = **f**iltration and removal of old blood cells and encapsulated micro-organisms

I = **i**mmunological functions (production of the immunoglobulin IgM and opsonins)

S = **s**torage function (30% of the total platelets within the spleen)

H= **h**aematopoiesis (in the developing fetus).

It has recently been found that the spleen has an endocrine function through the production of an immunopotentiating peptide called tuftsin.

The kidney, rather than the spleen, is the major site of erythropoietin secretion. Note that the spleen acts as a site of haematopoiesis in the adult only in diseased states where extramedullary haematopoiesis is a feature, such as thalassaemia.

Splenectomy (ie removal of the spleen) may be performed as an emergency procedure when the spleen has ruptured through trauma, or as an elective (ie scheduled) procedure, usually for haematological disorders where hypersplenism has caused an abnormality in one or more blood parameters. It is essential to understand the anatomical relations of the spleen (eg the pancreatic tail, stomach, splenic flexure of the colon, left kidney, diaphragm) in order to prevent inadvertent injury to these at splenectomy. Splenectomised patients are at high risk of postsplenectomy sepsis, especially from encapsulated organisms such as *Haemophilus* species, meningococci and streptococci. Prophylaxis consists of the relevant immunisations and lifelong penicillin.

45   D   Lies level with the hilum of the kidneys

The transpyloric plane (of Addison) is an important landmark. It lies halfway between the suprasternal notch and the symphysis pubis at the level of L1. It coincides with the following:

- L1 vertebra
- fundus of gallbladder
- hilum of kidneys
- hilum of spleen
- pylorus of the stomach (hence the name transpyloric)
- termination of the spinal cord in adults
- neck of pancreas
- origin of the portal vein
- origin of the superior (not the inferior) mesenteric artery
- duodenojejunal flexure
- attachment of transverse mesocolon
- tip of the ninth costal cartilage.

The aorta bifurcates at the level of L4, not L1.

46 D The anterior surface of the right adrenal gland is
        overlapped by the inferior vena cava

The adrenal glands lie anterosuperior to the upper part of each
kidney. They weigh approximately 5 g each and measure 50 mm
vertically, 30 mm across and 10 mm in thickness. They are
somewhat asymmetrical, with the right adrenal being pyramidal
in shape and the left crescentic; they lie within their own
compartments of the renal (Gerota's) fascia. A fascial septum
separates the adrenal gland from the kidney, which explains why
in nephrectomy (removal of the kidney) the adrenal gland is not
usually displaced (or even seen).

Each gland, although only weighing a few grams, has three
arteries supplying it: a direct branch from the aorta, a branch
from the renal artery and a branch from the inferior phrenic
artery. This reflects the high metabolic demands of the tissue.
The single main suprarenal vein drains into the nearest available
vessel; on the right it drains into the inferior vena cava and on
the left, directly into the renal vein. The right adrenal gland is
tucked medially behind the inferior vena cava. In addition, the
right suprarenal vein is particularly short and stubby. Both these
features make the inferior vena cava vulnerable to damage in a
right adrenalectomy.

The adrenal gland comprises an outer cortex and an inner
medulla, which represent two developmentally and functionally
independent endocrine glands within the same anatomical
structure. The medulla is derived from the neural crest
(ectoderm). It receives preganglionic sympathetic fibres from the
greater splanchnic nerve and secretes epinephrine or adrenaline
(70%) and norepinephrine or noradrenaline (30%). The cortex is
derived from mesoderm and consists of three layers or zones.

ANSWERS

Abdomen and pelvis – Answers

The layers from the surface inwards may be remembered by the mnemonic GFR (which is also the abbreviation for glomerular filtration rate):

G = zona **g**lomerulosa (secretes aldosterone)

F = zona **f**asciculata (secretes cortisol and sex steroids)

R = zona **r**eticularis (secretes cortisol and sex steroids).

 47 ▸ **D Is unimportant in humans**

The vermiform (worm-shaped) appendix is a blind-ending tube varying in length (commonly 6–9 cm), which opens into the posteromedial wall of the caecum, where the taeniae coli converge. The appendix is an intraperitoneal structure and therefore has its own short mesentery, the mesoappendix. Within the mesentery lies the appendicular artery, a branch of the ileocolic artery that arises from the superior mesenteric artery.

The surface marking of the base of the appendix is situated a third of the way up the line joining the anterosuperior iliac spine to the umbilicus (McBurney's point). This is an important landmark when performing an appendicectomy (McBurney's or gridiron) incision. The position of the free end of the appendix is, however, very variable. The most commonly found at surgery is the retrocaecal or retrocolic position (75% of cases), with the subcaecal or pelvic position next in order of frequency (20% of cases). Less commonly, in 5% of cases, it lies in the preileal or retro-ileal positions, in front of the caecum or in the right paracolic gutter.

The appendix has no known physiological function in humans and can therefore be removed with no consequences. It probably represents a degenerated portion of the caecum that, in ancestral forms, aided in cellulose digestion. In other animals, the appendix is much larger and provides a pouch off the main intestinal tract, in which cellulose can be trapped and subjected to prolonged digestion. The abundance of lymphoid tissue within the submucosa of the appendix has prompted the concept that the appendix is the human equivalent of the avian bursa of Fabricius, as a site of maturation of thymus-independent lymphocytes. Although no discernible change in immune function results from appendicectomy, the prominence of lymphatic tissue in the appendix of young adults seems important in its aetiology.

ANSWERS

Abdomen and pelvis – Answers

48   B   Can result in thrombosis of the appendicular artery
(endarteritis obliterans)

Acute appendicitis is the most common acute surgical condition
of the abdomen. About 7% of the population will have
appendicitis in their lifetime, with the peak incidence occurring
between the ages of 10 and 30 years. Appendicitis is relatively
uncommon at the two extremes of life because obstruction of
the lumen is the usual cause of appendicitis, and the lumen of
the appendix is relatively wide in the infant and frequently
completely obliterated in elderly people.

Afferent nerve fibres concerned with the conduction of visceral
pain from the appendix accompany the sympathetic nerves and
enter the spinal cord at the level of T10. Consequently, the
appendix refers visceral pain to the T10 dermatome that lies at
the level of the umbilicus. Only later, when the parietal
peritoneum overlying the appendix becomes inflamed, does the
pain become more intense and localise to the right iliac fossa in
the region of McBurney's point.

The following three factors contribute to why the appendix is
prone to infection:

1. It is a long, narrow, blind-ended tube that encourages stasis
   of large bowel contents.

2. It has a large amount of lymphoid tissue in its wall
   (submucosa).

3. The lumen has a tendency to become obstructed by
   hardened intestinal contents (enteroliths or faecoliths), which
   leads to further stagnation of its contents.

It is worth understanding the sequence of events underlying
acute appendicitis. The initial event is probably related to
obstruction of the mouth of the appendix. The most common

cause of obstruction is a faecolith. This leads to formation of a closed system and the build-up of mucinous secretions (appendiceal mucocele). The distended appendix can become secondarily infected and inflamed (appendicitis), and can subsequently lead to formation of an appendix mass or abscess. Alternatively, the pressure within this closed system may begin to rise until the point is reached when it starts to compress the superficial veins in the wall of the appendix. Obstruction to venous outflow leads to oedema and a further increase in pressure. The pressure continues to rise until eventually the appendiceal artery is compressed and it then thromboses (endarteritis obliterans). As the appendiceal artery is an end artery and does not anastomose with any other artery, it therefore represents the entire vascular supply of the appendix. The appendix subsequently undergoes ischaemic necrosis and gangrene, which may eventually result in a perforated appendix.

Acute appendicitis almost always requires surgical intervention. This may be performed by open or laparoscopic techniques. It rarely resolves with conservative management and 'watchful waiting' risks progression to perforation and generalised peritonitis, which carries with it a high mortality. There is only one situation in which conservative management is a feasible alternative to surgery and that is when an appendix mass (or abscess) is present and the patient is not compromised. Even then, however, it is advisable to remove the appendix later, after an interval of 6–8 weeks.

ANSWERS

49 ▸ D Provides a route of access to the lesser sac

The greater omentum (or gastrocolic omentum) is a double sheet of peritoneum, fused and folded on itself to form an integral structure made up of four layers. It contains adipose tissue of variable amounts, depending on the nutritional status of the patient, and hangs down like an apron overlying loops of intestine.

The anterior two layers descend from the greater curvature of the stomach (the lesser, not the greater, omentum arises from the lesser curvature of the stomach), where they are continuous with the peritoneum on the anterior and posterior surfaces of the stomach. Posteriorly, they ascend up to the transverse colon, where they loosely blend with the peritoneum on the anterior and posterior surfaces of the transverse colon and the transverse mesocolon above it.

The right and left gastroepiploic arteries run between the layers of the greater omentum and supply it, close to the greater curvature of the stomach. The greater omentum may undergo torsion and, if this is extensive, the blood supply to part of it may be cut off, causing necrosis. The lesser sac may be accessed through the greater omentum (by incising between the greater curvature of the stomach and the transverse colon and lifting the stomach up).

The greater omentum is of paramount surgical importance. Surgeons sometimes use the omentum to buttress an intestinal anastomosis, or in the closure of a perforated gastric or duodenal ulcer ('omental patch repair'). One important function of the greater omentum is to attempt to limit the spread of intraperitoneal infections. Indeed, the greater omentum is often referred to by surgeons as the 'great policeman of the abdomen'. The lower, right and left margins are free and it moves about the peritoneal cavity in response to peristaltic movements of the

ANSWERS

MCQs in Applied Basic Sciences for Medical Students: Volume 1

neighbouring gut. In an acutely inflamed appendix, for example, the inflammatory exudates cause the omentum to adhere to the appendix and wrap itself around the infected organ. By this means, the infection is often localised to a small area of the peritoneal cavity, thus saving the patient from a serious generalised peritonitis. The greater omentum is also commonly found plugging the neck of a hernial sac, thereby preventing the entry of coils of small intestine and strangulation of bowel. In the first 2 years of life, the greater omentum is poorly developed and thus is less protective in a young child.

50   B   Enter the bladder obliquely forming a flap valve

The ureters are segmental muscular tubes, 25 cm long, composed of smooth (involuntary) muscle throughout their entire length. They are lined by transitional epithelium (urothelium) also throughout their length. Indeed the whole urinary tract, including the renal pelvis and bladder, with the exception of the terminal urethra, is lined by transitional epithelium.

The clinical significance of this lining is that the whole urinary tract epithelium is susceptible to widespread malignant change in response to carcinogens and, as a result, tumours of the urothelium are more often multifocal compared with other sites (the so-called 'field effect'). Only the terminal urethra (its glandular part) is lined by stratified squamous epithelium.

It is important to recognise and distinguish the ureter from surrounding vessels and nerves in the living body during surgery in order to prevent inadvertent damage. The ureter is characteristically a whitish, non-pulsatile cord, which shows peristaltic activity when gently pinched with forceps (ie it vermiculates). There is no situation where it is more important to recognise and preserve the ureters than at hysterectomy, where the ureters lie in close proximity to the uterine vessels and ligaments. Incorrect ligation of the ureters instead of the uterine vessels may be prevented by correctly identifying the ureters (through assessment for vermiculation) and remembering the mnemonic 'water under the bridge' (ie the ureters are crossed above by the uterine arteries).

Blood supply to the ureters, as in the oesophagus, is segmental. The upper third is supplied by the renal arteries, the middle third from branches given off from the descending abdominal aorta and the lower third by the superior and inferior vesical arteries. Blood supply to the middle third is the most tenuous. Consequently, the middle third of the ureter is most vulnerable to postoperative ischaemia and stricture formation if its blood supply is endangered by stripping the ureter clean of its surrounding tissue at surgery.

Along the course of the ureter there are three constrictions that are worth remembering because they are often the site of hold-up for ureteric calculi (stones):

1. Pelviureteric junction

2. Where the ureter crosses the pelvic brim in the region of the bifurcation of the common iliac artery

3. Vesicoureteric junction.

The last is the point of narrowest calibre. In both sexes the ureters run obliquely through the bladder wall for 1–2 cm before reaching their orifices at the upper lateral angles of the trigone. This forms a flap valve that prevents reflux of urine retrogradely back up the ureters. If this flap valve is congenitally deficient, vesicoureteric reflux results.

51 ▶ D Contains the pampiniform plexus

The contents of the spermatic cord are easily remembered using the 'rule of 3s':

- Three constituents: vas deferens (the round ligament is the female equivalent), lymphatics, obliterated processus vaginalis.

- Three nerves: genital branch of the genitofemoral nerve (motor to cremaster, sensory to cord), ilioinguinal nerve (within the inguinal canal but outside the spermatic cord), autonomics.

- Three arteries: testicular artery, artery to the vas (from the superior or inferior vesical artery), cremasteric artery (from the inferior epigastric artery).

- Three veins: pampiniform plexus, vein from the vas, cremasteric vein.

- Three fascial coverings: internal spermatic fascia, external spermatic fascia, cremasteric muscle and fascia (not the dartos muscle, which is contained within the wall of the scrotum).

ANSWERS

Abdomen and pelvis – Answers

52   D   Is supplied by T10 sympathetic nerves

The testis is supplied by the testicular artery, which arises directly from the descending abdominal aorta at about the level of L2. Although at first glance this may seem illogical, when the testis is in closer proximity to other blood vessels such as the internal iliac, the explanation lies in the fact that the testis develops high up on the posterior abdominal wall early in embryonic life.

As it descends into the scrotum during development, the testis carries with it the same blood supply that it received when it was positioned on the posterior abdominal wall (ie from the aorta).

The testis drains by way of the pampiniform plexus into the inferior vena cava on the right side, but into the left renal vein on the left. This may account for the fact that varicoceles (varicosities of the pampiniform plexus secondary to incompetent venous valves) are more common on the left compared with the right. The accumulation of serous fluid around the testis is known as a hydrocele.

As a general rule with regard to lymphatic drainage, superficial lymphatics (ie in subcutaneous tissues) tend to run with superficial veins, whereas deep lymphatics run with arteries. The testis thus drains lymph to the para-aortic set of lymph nodes, because the testicular artery arises from the aorta. The testis never drains to the inguinal group of lymph nodes, although the scrotum may. The clinical consequence of this is that a testicular carcinoma never results in inguinal lymphadenopathy, unless the scrotum is also involved. A scrotal carcinoma, on the other hand, would be expected to produce inguinal lymphadenopathy and this holds true in clinical practice.

The testis is supplied by T10 sympathetic nerves. The consequences of this are twofold: first, it results in testicular pain (trauma, testicular torsion, etc.) being referred to the umbilicus

ANSWERS

MCQs in Applied Basic Sciences for Medical Students: Volume 1

(T10 dermatome); and, second, the ureters are also supplied by T10 sympathetics. Thus, a renal calculus may refer pain down to the testis, as is seen in classic renal colic.

B Lies medial to the obdurator nerve and anterior to the ureter

The ovary is ovoid in shape, measuring about $3 \times 2 \times 1$ cm (smaller than the testis), being smaller before menarche and postmenopausally. The anterior border of the ovary is attached to the posterior leaf of the broad ligament by a double fold of peritoneum, the mesovarium. The ovary is thus an intraperitoneal structure and the surface of the ovary, covered with cuboidal epithelium, faces the peritoneal cavity, so ova extruded from the ovary actually pass into the peritoneal cavity. One consequence of this is that an ectopic pregnancy may occur within the peritoneal cavity, in addition to within the fallopian tube.

The ovary flops laterally to lie in the ovarian fossa on the lateral pelvic wall. Immediately behind the fossa is the ureter, which may be damaged while operating on the ovary, and lateral to the ovary is the obturator neurovascular bundle. A diseased ovary may therefore cause referred pain along the cutaneous distribution of the obturator nerve on the inner side of the thigh. Nerve supply to the ovary is sympathetic, originating at T10, and therefore ovarian pain may also be referred to the periumbilical region.

The suspensory ligament of the ovary transmits the ovarian artery, vein and lymphatics. As a general rule, the superficial lymphatics (ie in subcutaneous tissues) tend to run with the superficial veins, whereas the deep lymphatics run with the arteries. As the artery starts from the aorta, lymph drainage therefore passes to the para-aortic lymph nodes. The same applies for the testis in the male.

54 ▶ A Is drained by tributaries of both inferior mesenteric and internal iliac veins

The rectum is 12 cm long, starting at the level of S3 and ending at the puborectalis (levator ani/pelvic floor). It is lined by typical columnar intestinal epithelium with many mucus-secreting cells (transitional epithelium is almost exclusively confined to the urinary tract of mammals, where it is highly specialised to accommodate a great deal of stretch and to withstand the toxicity of the urine).

The rectum has no mesentery and is therefore regarded as retroperitoneal. It is covered by peritoneum on its front and sides in its upper third, only on its front in its middle third and the rectum lies below the peritoneal reflection in its lower third. Do not be confused; although the rectum has no mesentery, the visceral pelvic fascia around the rectum is often referred to by surgeons as the mesorectum. The pararectal lymph nodes are found within the mesorectum, which is removed together with the rectum as a package during rectal excision for carcinoma.

Blood supply is by way of the superior rectal (inferior mesenteric), middle rectal (internal iliac) and inferior rectal (internal pudendal) arteries. The importance of understanding the blood supply of the rectum lies in its vulnerability during the resection of a rectal carcinoma and the formation of a join (anastomosis) from the two remaining ends of bowel. If the blood supply to the anastomosis is tenuous, then the anastomosis may break down in the postoperative period with disastrous consequences. The venous drainage is as for the arteries. Note, however, that there is a portosystemic anastomosis in the lower rectal and upper anal canal walls, as branches of the superior rectal (portal) and inferior/middle rectal veins (systemic) meet in the external and internal venous plexus. This creates a site where haemorrhoids may form in portal hypertension.

The rectum receives parasympathetic fibres from the pelvic splanchnic nerves, or nervi erigentes, originating from S2–4. It functions to relax the internal sphincter, contract the bowel and transmit a sense of fullness. Note that the vagus nerve supplies bowel only up to two-thirds of the way along the transverse colon. The whole of the rest of the bowel inferior to this level (the so-called hindgut) receives parasympathetic fibres by way of the pelvic splanchnic nerves. Remember that parasympathetic outflow from the spinal cord is craniosacral, whereas sympathetic outflow is thoracolumbar. Sympathetic supply to the rectum is through the lumbar splanchnics and superior hypogastric plexus. Sympathetics contract the internal sphincter, relax the bowel and transmit pain.

55   **E   The ureter is closely related to the lateral fornix of the cervix**

The supports of the uterus are extremely important. The lateral (or transverse) cervical ligaments condense around the uterine artery and run to the lateral pelvic wall. The uterosacral ligaments are primarily condensations of fascia running backwards from the cervix of the uterus, past the rectum and attaching to the sacrum. The round ligament of the uterus is the female remnant of the embryonic gubernaculum, which guides the testis to the scrotum in the male.

The continuation of the ovarian ligament is in the broad ligament attaching the ovary to the uterus. The round ligament continues from the wall of the uterus in the anterior leaf of the broad ligament to the pelvic wall and then through the deep inguinal ring and inguinal canal, to fade out into the labium majorum. It is important only to help hold the uterus in its usual anteverted, anteflexed position (ie the uterus tends to lie tipped forwards over the female bladder).

Some support is also offered by the anterior pubocervical ligaments. Similarly, the broad ligament holds the uterus in that position, but does not contribute a great deal to preventing uterine prolapse (procidentia). The latter is a condition where the pelvic floor is so weakened, usually after multiple childbirths, that the uterus tends to prolapse through the vagina. This can adversely affect the base of the bladder or even obstruct the ureters and can therefore lead to urinary infections, incontinence and renal failure.

The blood supply comes mainly from the uterine artery, which takes a very tortuous course up the uterus (to allow for expansion in uterine hypertrophy, eg pregnancy). It is a branch of the internal iliac. When it reaches the uterus, the uterine artery must pass across and above the ureter which is heading past the uterus to the bladder. During hysterectomy, this relationship is enormously important because the uterine arteries must be ligated and cut. Clearly one must recognise the difference and realise the close proximity of the ureters and uterine arteries.

The ureters lie adjacent to the lateral fornix of the cervix. Consequently, a ureteric calculus may be felt in the lateral fornix on vaginal examination. The posterior fornix actually has the peritoneum of the rectouterine pouch of Douglas overlying it; this is normally occupied by coils of small intestine or sigmoid colon and lies between the uterus anteriorly and the rectum posteriorly. The rectouterine pouch of Douglas is the most dependent part of the pelvis. Consequently blood may collect here in a ruptured ectopic pregnancy. A needle may be passed into this space (in an attempt to aspirate blood) in order to diagnose the condition (culdocentesis). Furthermore, the instrument used in illegal abortions, if it misses the cavity of the uterus, could actually penetrate the posterior fornix and subsequently the peritoneal cavity, often leading to fatal peritonitis and sepsis.

D The gastroduodenal artery is a branch of the common hepatic artery

The blood supply of the stomach is initially quite confusing, easily forgotten and commonly asked about, but a few key rules make this a simple area of anatomy that will never be forgotten.

Rule 1

The coeliac trunk divides into three main branches, which can be easily remembered by the mnemonic left hand side (LHS):

L = **l**eft gastric artery

H = common **h**epatic artery

S = **s**plenic artery.

Rule 2

For the purposes of remembering the blood supply to the stomach, the stomach can be divided into three main areas:

1 = lesser curvature

2 = greater curvature

3 = fundus.

Rule 3

The lesser curvature is supplied by the left and right gastric arteries. The left gastric artery, as already mentioned, comes directly off the coeliac trunk. The right gastric artery is a branch of the common hepatic artery.

ANSWERS

Abdomen and pelvis – Answers

Rule 4

The greater curvature is supplied by the right and left gastroepiploic arteries. The right gastroepiploic artery comes off the gastroduodenal artery and the left artery off the splenic artery.

Rule 5

The fundus is supplied by the six, or so, short gastric arteries that arise from the splenic artery.

Rule 6

The gastroduodenal artery is an important artery to remember for clinical purposes. It arises from the common hepatic artery and lies posterior to the first part of the duodenum. A posteriorly sited duodenal ulcer may erode through the duodenal wall into the blood vessel, causing catastrophic, life-threatening haemorrhage. Urgent endoscopy or laparotomy may be required to stop the bleeding.

Upper and lower limbs
Answers

57   E   Cloquet's node lies more medially within the femoral canal

The boundaries of the femoral triangle are the inguinal ligament superiorly, the medial border of adductor longus medially and the medial border of sartorius laterally.

The contents of the femoral triangle from lateral to medial may be easily remembered by the mnemonic NAVY:

N = **n**erve (femoral) outside the femoral sheath

A = **a**rtery (femoral) within the femoral sheath

V = **v**ein (femoral) within the femoral sheath

Y = **Y** fronts (mostly medially).

Within the femoral sheath lie the femoral artery, vein and a space known as the femoral canal. The purpose of the femoral canal is to allow the laterally placed femoral vein to expand into it, thereby encouraging venous return. However, a piece of bowel or omentum may extend down into the femoral space, causing a femoral hernia. Within the space of the femoral canal there normally lies extraperitoneal fat and a lymph node that is often given its eponymous name, Cloquet's lymph node. Cloquet's lymph node drains the lower limb, perineum and anterior abdominal wall inferior to the umbilicus. It may be enlarged (as in inguinal lymphadenopathy) in cases of carcinoma and infection at these sites.

The femoral artery lies at the mid-inguinal point (halfway between the anterior superior iliac spine and symphysis pubis), as opposed to the mid-point of the inguinal ligament (halfway between the anterior superior iliac spine and pubic tubercle), which is the surface marking of the deep inguinal ring. The surface marking of the femoral artery is imperative to understand because not only does it provide a site for the clinician to assess the femoral pulse, but it also provides the clinician with a surface landmark for gaining access to the femoral artery for procedures such as coronary angioplasty and lower limb angiography and embolectomy.

58   ▶   B   Has high mobility at the expense of stability

The shoulder joint, similar to the hip joint, is a synovial joint of the ball-and-socket variety. The joint cavity, as is the case with all synovial joints, is lined by articular hyaline cartilage and not fibrocartilage. Again as with all joints, stability is brought about by the way the various bones articulate with each other (through their incongruous surfaces) and via the various ligaments, tendons and muscles that surround the joint.

Clearly, it is impossible to have a joint that is both highly mobile and perfectly stabile, because a highly mobile joint requires a wide range of movement, in all possible degrees of freedom, which is in itself intrinsically unstable. In contrast to the hip joint, where stability is of paramount importance, in the shoulder joint mobility comes at the expense of stability.

The rotator cuff muscles are the most important factor in maintaining the stability of the shoulder joint and preventing dislocation. The ligaments and bones are less important in the case of the shoulder joint. There are only four muscles of the rotator cuff, which can be remembered by the mnemonic SITS:

S = **s**upraspinatus

I = **i**nfraspinatus

T = **t**eres minor

S = **s**ubscapularis.

Note that teres major is not a rotator cuff muscle, and also that the first three muscles are placed posteriorly, behind the shoulder joint, whereas only one of the rotator cuff muscles (subscapularis) is positioned anteriorly. This could partly explain why the shoulder more commonly dislocates anteriorly rather than posteriorly. An alternative explanation may relate to the deficiency of the joint capsule inferiorly, which makes the shoulder susceptible to anteroinferior dislocation while in the abducted, externally rotated position. These two explanations are not mutually exclusive.

It should never be forgotten that the axillary nerve lies in close proximity to the shoulder joint and the surgical neck of the humerus. Consequently, it is vulnerable to injury at the time of a shoulder dislocation, or while attempting to reduce the shoulder back into its normal position after a dislocation. It is therefore imperative (from both a clinical and a medicolegal point of view) that the integrity of the axillary nerve be documented, both after seeing the patient who has a dislocated shoulder and after a successful reduction.

59

B The hip joint can refer pain to the knee

The hip joint, like the shoulder joint, is a synovial joint of the ball-and-socket variety. In general it can be said that, in all joints, stability and range of movement are inversely proportional to each other.

The shoulder joint is the most commonly dislocated joint in the body because it has adapted to a high degree of mobility at the expense of stability. The hip joint is an exception to the rule and provides a remarkable example of a joint that has a high degree of both mobility and stability. Its stability largely results from the adaptation of the acetabulum and femoral head to each other, with a snug fit of the femoral head into the acetabulum, deepened by the labrum and further reinforced by three ligaments on the outside of the capsule: the iliofemoral, ischiofemoral and pubofemoral ligaments. The iliofemoral ligament (of Bigelow) is the strongest of the three ligaments. The short muscles of the gluteal region are important muscular stabilisers.

As the hip is such a stable joint, it requires considerable force to become dislocated. When it does, the hip joint usually dislocates in the setting of a road traffic accident, where it typically dislocates posteriorly. The hip's great range of mobility results from the femur having a long neck that is much narrower than its head.

The hip joint lies deep to the pulsation of the femoral artery at the mid-inguinal point (halfway between the anterosuperior iliac spine and symphysis pubis, in contrast to the middle of the inguinal ligament, which is halfway between the anterosuperior iliac spine and pubic tubercle, marking the site of the deep inguinal ring). The mid-inguinal point is the surface marking of the hip joint so pain at this point may indicate pathology originating in the hip joint. Posterior to the hip lies the important sciatic nerve. Consequently, the sciatic nerve is at risk in a posterior surgical approach to the hip, or in a posterior dislocation.

The hip joint is innervated by the sciatic, femoral and obturator nerves (Hilton's law), which also innervate the knee joint. This may explain why hip pathology commonly refers pain to the knee. In a child who presents with a painful knee, examination should always include the ipsilateral hip joint, in addition to the knee, so as not to miss a diseased hip.

The blood supply to the femoral head originates from three important sources:

1. Most importantly, via retinacular vessels that run up from the trochanteric anastomosis and then along the neck of the femur to supply the major part of the head. The trochanteric anastomosis is formed by an anastomosis of the medial and lateral circumflex femoral arteries and the superior and inferior gluteal arteries.

2. From the obturator artery in the ligamentum teres (round ligament) – usually more important in the young child.

3. Via the nutrient, or diaphyseal, artery of the femur, originating from the profunda femoris artery.

A fracture of the neck of the femur may disrupt these vessels and consequently disrupt the blood flow to the femoral head, resulting in avascular necrosis. This condition frequently occurs in old women who have osteoporosis after a fall. The femoral head must be taken out and replaced with a prosthesis quickly, so that mobility may be regained.

60

E The pulsation of the radical artery may be felt at its base

The contents and boundaries of the anatomical snuffbox are as follows:

Base:
From proximal to distal: radial styloid, scaphoid, trapezium, base of first metacarpal.

Roof:
Skin
Fascia.

Medially (ulnar side):
Extensor pollicis longus tendon.

Laterally (radial side):
Extensor pollicis brevis tendon
Abductor pollicis longus tendon.

Contents:
Cephalic vein (beginning in its roof)
Terminal branches of radial nerve (supplying the overlying skin)
Radial artery (on its floor).

The anatomical snuffbox is clinically an important region for three reasons: first, tenderness within the anatomical snuffbox may indicate a fractured scaphoid bone. This is important to recognise because radiographs are often unremarkable in the early stages and, if left untreated, there is a risk of avascular necrosis of the scaphoid (in fact the proximal scaphoid segment necroses because it receives its blood supply from distal to proximal). Second, tendonitis of the tendons of abductor pollicis longus and extensor pollicis brevis may occur; this is known as

DeQuervain's tenovaginitis stenosans. Third, the cephalic vein is almost invariably found in the region of the anatomical snuffbox, which therefore forms a useful landmark for the purpose of gaining intravenous access.

61 C The suprapatellar bursa (pouch) communicates with the knee joint

The knee joint is a synovial joint (the largest in the body) of the modified hinge variety. The bony contours contribute little to the stability of the joint. Nevertheless, the ligaments and muscles make it a very stable joint that rarely dislocates.

The cruciate ligaments are two very strong ligaments that cross each other within the joint cavity, but are excluded from the synovial cavity by a covering of synovial membrane (they are therefore described as being intracapsular, but extrasynovial). They are crucial in the sense that they are essential for stability of the knee. They are named anterior and posterior according to their tibial attachments. Thus the anterior cruciate ligament is attached to the anterior intercondylar area of the tibia and runs upwards, backwards and laterally to attach itself to the medial surface of the lateral femoral condyle. The anterior cruciate prevents anterior displacement of the tibia on the femur. Backward displacement of the tibia on the femur is prevented by the stronger posterior cruciate ligament, so the integrity of the latter is therefore important when walking downstairs or downhill. Tears of the anterior cruciate ligament are common in sports injuries; tears of the posterior cruciate ligament, however, are rare because it is much stronger than the anterior cruciate.

Bursae are lubricating devices found wherever skin, muscle or tendon rubs against bone. There are about a dozen bursae related to the knee joint. The details are not important, only the salient points, eg it would be important to remember that the suprapatellar bursa communicates with the knee joint. An effusion of the knee may therefore extend some three to four fingerbreadths above the patella into the suprapatellar pouch. The prepatellar and infrapatellar bursae do not communicate with the knee joint, but may become inflamed, causing a painful bursitis. Inflammation of the prepatellar bursa is known as housemaid's knee, whereas that of the infrapatellar bursa is called clergyman's knee.

The menisci, or semilunar cartilages, are crescent-shaped laminae of fibrocartilage, the medial being larger and less curved than the lateral. They have an important role in:

- distributing the load by increasing the congruity of the articulation
- contributing to stability of the knee by their physical presence and by acting as providers of proprioceptive feedback
- acting as shock absorbers through a 'cushioning' effect
- probably assisting in lubrication.

The menisci do not, however, play a role in the locking/unlocking mechanism of the knee joint. This is primarily the responsibility of the popliteus muscle.

The menisci are liable to injury from twisting strains applied to a flexed weight-bearing knee. The medial meniscus is much less mobile than the lateral meniscus (because of its strong attachment to the medial collateral ligament of the knee joint) and it cannot as easily accommodate abnormal stresses placed upon it. This, in part, explains why meniscal lesions are much more common on the medial than on the lateral side.

The menisci are so effective that, if they are removed, the force taken by the articular hyaline cartilage during peak loading increases by about fivefold. Meniscectomy (removal of the menisci), or damage to the menisci, therefore exposes the articular hyaline cartilage to much greater forces than normal and evidence of degenerative osteoarthritis is seen in 75% of patients 10 years after meniscectomy.

62   E   Roots lie in the neck between the scalenus anterior and medius muscles

There are two principal enlargements of the spinal cord, the cervical and lumbar enlargements, that give rise to the brachial and lumbrosacral plexus, respectively, which innervate the upper and lower limbs. Both enlargements are caused by the greatly increased mass of motor cells in the anterior horns of grey matter in these situations.

The brachial plexus has root values in C5–8 and T1. In 10% of cases the brachial plexus may be either pre-fixed (C4–8) or post-fixed (C6–T2) as an anatomical variant.

The anatomical relations of the different parts of the brachial plexus are important:

Roots: exit their respective intervertebral foraminae between the scalenus anterior and medius muscles (interscalene space).

Trunks: at the base of the posterior triangle of the neck, lying on the first rib posterior to the third part of the subclavian artery.

Divisions: behind the middle third of the clavicle.

Cords: in the axilla, in intimate relation with the second part of the axillary artery.

Terminal branches: in relation with the third part of the axillary artery.

The relation of the roots, trunks and divisions of the brachial plexus to the scalene muscles, first rib and clavicle is important.

ANSWERS

Upper and lower limb – Answers

Compression within a fixed space (the thoracic outlet) may lead to symptoms resulting from compression of the brachial plexus and/or nearby vascular structures (subclavian artery and vein). This is known as the thoracic outlet syndrome.

The serratus anterior muscle is innervated by the long thoracic nerve of Bell (C5, C6, C7). This may be remembered by the old aphorism 'C5, C6, C7, Bell's of heaven'. Denervation of the serratus muscle may result in winging of the scapula.

There are two recognised types of brachial plexus palsy; both usually occur as a result of trauma or obstetric injury. The first follows injury to the upper roots of the brachial plexus (typically C5–7) and is known as the Erb–Duchenne palsy. The arm typically lies in a waiter's tip position. The second follows injury to the lower roots of the brachial plexus (typically C8, T1) and is known as Klumpke's palsy. The hand in this case typically takes on the position of a 'clawed' hand.

63 ▶ C The musculocutaneous nerve arises from the lateral cord

This is a common question! The three cords of the brachial plexus lie in close relation to the second part of the axillary artery. Thus, the posterior, lateral and medial cords lie posteriorly, laterally and medially to the second part of the axillary artery, respectively, in the axilla. There is no anterior cord:

Lateral cord: musculocutaneous nerve

Medial cord: ulnar nerve

Posterior cord: radial nerve, axillary nerve

Medial and lateral cords: median nerve.

D Contains 10 tendons within it

The carpal tunnel is a fibro-osseous tunnel situated on the flexor aspect of the proximal part of the hand and lying between the flexor retinaculum and the carpal bones. It contains the median nerve and 10 flexor tendons, including:

- four tendons of flexor digitorum superficialis

- four tendons of flexor digitorum profundus

- flexor carpi radialis tendon

- flexor pollicis longus tendon.

The flexor retinaculum is attached to the tubercle of the scaphoid and pisiform proximally and the hook of the hamate and trapezium distally. Its function is to prevent bow stringing of the flexor tendons at the wrist.

As the carpal tunnel exists as a confined space, entrapment of the median nerve may occur within it. This is commonly caused by a build-up of fluid within the carpal tunnel or hypertrophy of the bones/ligaments/tendons that surround, or are contained within, the carpal tunnel. Compression of the median nerve within the carpal tunnel is known as carpal tunnel syndrome. Note that this is different from the cubital tunnel syndrome, which refers to compression of the ulnar nerve behind the medial epicondyle at the elbow. The ulnar artery and nerve do not pass through the carpal tunnel, but instead pass superficial to the carpal tunnel in their own fibro-osseous tunnel, commonly given the name Guyon's canal. The ulnar nerve and artery are therefore unaffected in carpal tunnel syndrome.

The clinical features of carpal tunnel syndrome relate to loss of function of the median nerve. There are both motor and sensory components. The median nerve supplies four muscles in the hand, given by the mnemonic LOAF:

ANSWERS

Upper and lower limb – Answers

L = **l**ateral two lumbricals

O = **o**pponens pollicis

A = **a**bductor pollicis brevis

F = **f**lexor pollicis brevis.

All four muscles are weak in someone with carpal tunnel syndrome. In addition, there is loss of sensation over the lateral three and a half digits, which is median nerve territory. However, as the palmar cutaneous branch of the median nerve passes superficial to the carpal tunnel, there is no loss of sensation over the thenar eminence in someone who has carpal tunnel syndrome.

65 ▶ **E** The dorsalis pedis pulse is lateral to the extensor hallucis logues tendon

The arterial supply to the lower limb is important because atherosclerosis within the arteries can lead to peripheral vascular disease and symptoms of intermittent claudication. To determine the level of arterial obstruction, it is necessary to be able to palpate the pulses of the various parts of the arterial tree, which requires a precise knowledge of anatomy.

The aorta bifurcates into the common iliac vessels at the level of L4. The common iliac bifurcates into the external and internal iliac vessels. As the external iliac artery passes under the inguinal ligament, it changes its name to the common femoral artery. Thus, the femoral artery is a direct continuation of the external iliac artery. The pulsation of the femoral artery may be palpated at the mid-inguinal point (at a point halfway between the anterosuperior iliac spine and symphysis pubis). This is different to the mid-point of the inguinal ligament, which corresponds to a point halfway along the inguinal ligament (between the anterosuperior iliac spine and pubic tubercle), which in turn marks the site of the deep inguinal ring.

The common femoral artery divides 3–4 cm below the inguinal ligament, into superficial femoral and deep femoral (profunda femoris) branches. The superficial femoral artery is the most common site for peripheral vascular disease in the lower limb. The superficial femoral artery continues through the adductor canal (also known as the subsartorial or Hunter's canal) and, after passing through the adductor hiatus becomes known as the popliteal artery. Within the popliteal fossa, the popliteal artery lies deep to the tibial nerve and popliteal vein. This explains why a normal popliteal artery is so difficult to feel. A palpable popliteal artery normally implies that it is aneurysmal (abnormally dilated).

The popliteal artery bifurcates into anterior and posterior tibial arteries. The posterior tibial artery is easily palpated posterior to the medial malleolus at the level of the ankle. A useful mnemonic for remembering the order of structures behind the medial malleolus (from anterior to posterior) is 'Tom, Dick and Harry':

Tom = **t**ibialis posterior tendon (mostly anteriorly)

Dick = flexor **d**igitorum longus tendon

and = **a**rtery (posterior tibial), **n**erve (tibial nerve)

Harry = flexor **h**allucis longus tendon (mostly posteriorly).

The anterior tibial artery continues down into the foot as the dorsalis pedis artery. However, in 10% of individuals this is absent. The pulsation of dorsalis pedis may be felt lateral to the extensor hallucis longus tendon, between the first and second metatarsals. A useful mnemonic for remembering the order of structures in the anterior compartment of the leg (from medial to lateral) is:

'Tim, Hath A Very Nasty Disease, Parathyroid'

Tim = **t**ibialis anterior tendon (mostly medially)

Hath = extensor **h**allucis longus tendon

A Very Nasty = neurovascular bundle consisting of **a**rtery (dorsalis pedis), **v**eins (venae comitantes of anterior tibial) and **n**erve (deep peroneal nerve)

Disease = extensor **d**igitorum longus tendon

Parathyroid = **p**eroneus tertius tendon (mostly laterally).

66   A The cephalic vein lies within the deltopectoral groove

The superficial venous drainage of the upper and lower extremities forms an important piece of applied anatomy. There are four veins that the student should know well: the cephalic and basilic veins in the upper limb and the long and short saphenous veins in the lower limb. All run from superficial to deep and contain valves within their lumina. Both these factors prevent the reflux of blood and encourage venous return to the heart.

The cephalic vein of the upper limb starts in the roof of the anatomical snuffbox and runs up the lateral border of the arm. It lies within the groove between the deltoid and pectoralis major muscles (the deltopectoral groove) and ends by piercing the clavipectoral fascia to enter the axillary vein.

The basilic vein runs up the medial border of the upper limb. It perforates the deep fascia in the middle of the arm, halfway between the elbow and axilla, and becomes the axillary vein at the lower border of teres major.

The long (great) saphenous vein, the longest vein in the body, starts as the upward continuation of the medial marginal vein of the foot. It courses upwards in front of the medial malleolus, in close proximity to the saphenous nerve, and runs up to lie a hand's breadth behind the medial border of the patella. It ends by passing through the cribriform fascia that covers the saphenous opening of the fascia lata. Here it joins the femoral vein at the saphenofemoral junction.

The long saphenous vein is important clinically for three reasons:

1. Incompetence of the valves within it may lead to the formation of superficial venous dilatations in the distribution of the long saphenous vein. These are known as varicose veins.

2. As the anatomy of the long saphenous vein is so reliable (more so than any other vein in the body), it makes the long saphenous vein a good choice for a venous cut-down, if emergency venous access is required.

3. As a result of its remarkably constant anatomy and because the long saphenous vein is the longest vein in the body, it is often harvested in vascular surgery and used to bypass arterial obstructions, a good example being in the case of coronary artery bypass grafting procedures where the long saphenous vein is one of many grafts that may be used to bypass blocked coronary arteries.

The short (small) saphenous vein drains the lateral margin of the foot and lies with the sural nerve behind the lateral malleolus. It passes upwards in the subcutaneous fat to the midline of the calf, and pierces the deep fascia to enter the popliteal vein at the saphenopopliteal junction. Similar to the long saphenous vein, the short saphenous vein is vulnerable to the formation of varicose veins.

A number of tributaries join the great saphenous vein in the region of the saphenous opening. This is important for two reasons: first, they may form a site for recurrence after varicose vein surgery and, second, the fact that the upper end of the long saphenous vein has these tributaries converging upon it easily distinguishes it from the femoral vein, which at this level receives only the long saphenous vein itself. It is imperative that the long saphenous vein be distinguished from the femoral vein at the saphenofemoral junction, during varicose vein surgery, in order to prevent inadvertent ligation of the femoral vein, which one hears about from time to time in medicolegal reports.

If surgery is performed for varicose veins (a high ligation tie and stripping of the vein), the saphenous nerve (a branch of the femoral nerve) is vulnerable to injury when stripping the long saphenous vein, because of its close proximity to this vein. Likewise, the sural nerve is at risk of being injured when stripping the short saphenous vein.

The basic action of the interossei and lumbrical muscles is to cause extension at the interphalangeal joints and flexion at the metacarpophalangeal joints. In addition, the palmar interossei adduct (PAD) the fingers, whereas the dorsal interossei abduct (DAB) the fingers. The lateral two lumbricals are supplied by the median nerve and the medial two lumbricals by the ulnar nerve, although all the interossei are supplied by the ulnar nerve.

As a general rule all the intrinsic muscles of the hand are supplied by the ulnar nerve (T1), except for the LOAF muscles (lateral two lumbricals, opponens pollicis, abductor pollicis brevis and flexor pollicis brevis muscles).

The hand receives a rich arterial supply from both the radial and the ulnar arteries. In the palm they anastomose to form two palmar arterial arcades, the superficial and deep palmar arches. The superficial palmar arch is formed by a direct continuation of the ulnar artery meeting the superficial palmar branch of the radial artery. The deep palmar arch is an arterial arcade formed by the terminal branch of the radial artery anastomosing with the deep branch of the ulnar artery. For a visual assessment of the contribution of the radial and ulnar arteries to the blood supply of the hand, Allen's test may be performed. This involves making a clenched fist and occluding the radial and ulnar arteries. When the fist is released the skin of the palm is seen to be pale, although colour should return rapidly on the release of either one of the arteries. If there is an obvious delay after releasing the ulnar compared with the radial artery, it suggests that the radial supply is dominant and that procedures that could damage the radial artery (such as cannulation) should be avoided.

The deep fascia of the palm is known as the palmar aponeurosis. It is continuous proximally with the flexor retinaculum and widens distally in the hand by dividing into four slips, one for each finger.

The palmar aponeurosis is firmly attached to the skin of the palm and assists the latter in gripping an object. Also, by virtue of its toughness, it protects the underlying tendons and synovial sheaths. Contracture of the palmar aponeurosis and its digital slips may occur, resulting in fixed flexion deformities of the fingers concerned (usually the ring and little fingers). This is known as Dupuytren's contracture. Dupuytren's contracture is a phenomenon of the palmar aponeurosis and has nothing to do with the underlying muscles or tendons. Ischaemic contracture of muscle is known instead as Volkmann's ischaemic contracture, and usually results from an arterial injury, as a complication of a fracture or after compartment syndrome. It is caused by the replacement of muscle by fibrous tissue, which contracts to produce a deformity.

SECTION B
Applied Physiology

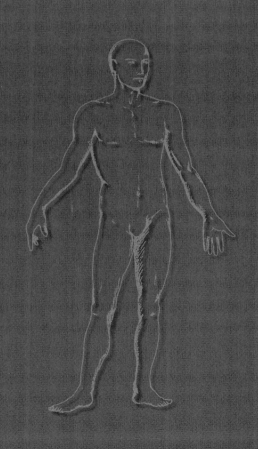

Nerve, muscle and neuroscience Questions

68 With regard to phototransduction:

○ A Photoreceptors depolarise in response to light exposure
○ B Phototransduction is a vitamin D-dependent process
○ C Upon exposure to light, cGMP levels within the photoreceptor fall
○ D Opening of cGMP-gated cation channels occurs in response to light
○ E Light photons are absorbed by transducin

69 With regard to visual field pathways:

○ A The axons contained within the optic nerve are derived from photoreceptors
○ B The optic tracts synapse in the medial geniculate nucleus of the thalamus
○ C Decussation is complete at the optic chiasma
○ D The macular region is grossly over-represented in the visual cortex
○ E Compression at the optic chiasma results in a homonymous hemianopia

70 ▶ Concerning the organisation of the cerebral cortex:

◯ A The right cerebral hemisphere is normally dominant

◯ B The primary visual cortex is located within the Brodmann area 17

◯ C The primary auditory cortex is located within Broca's area

◯ D The primary motor cortex is located within the postcentral gyrus

◯ E The primary somatosensory cortex is located within the precentral gyrus

71 ▶ Cerebrospinal fluid (CSF):

◯ A Is produced by arachnoid granulations

◯ B Is produced at a rate of 30 mL/min

◯ C Is situated within the subdural space

◯ D Flows between the lateral ventricles and the third ventricle via the foramen of Magendie

◯ E Turns over approximately four to five times daily

72 ▶ With regard to the composition of cerebrospinal fluid (CSF):

○ A CSF is produced through a passive process
○ B The composition of the CSF is identical to plasma
○ C The protein content of the CSF is 0.5% that of plasma
○ D The potassium content of the CSF is higher than that of plasma
○ E The pH of the CSF is heavily buffered

73 ▶ The speed of nerve conduction decreases with:

○ A Increasing axonal diameter
○ B Increasing membrane capacitance
○ C Decreasing axonal resistance
○ D Myelination by Schwann cells
○ E Increasing temperature

74 ▶ Skeletal muscle fibres:

○ A Are each normally innervated by more than one motor neuron

○ B Become less excitable as the extracellular levels of ionised calcium fall

○ C Take up calcium by the sarcotubular system when they contract

○ D Have actin and myosin filaments that shorten when the fibres contract

○ E Contain intracellular stores of calcium ions

75 ▶ With regard to nerve fibres:

○ A Impulses can travel in one direction only

○ B Nerve fibres continue to conduct impulses when extracellular sodium is replaced by potassium

○ C An action potential has an amplitude that varies directly with the strength of the stimulus

○ D The equilibrium potential for an ion species depends on the ratio of the concentrations of the ion outside and inside the cell

○ E Resting nerve cell membranes are more permeable to Na^+ than to K^+

76 ► With regard to smooth (visceral) muscle:

○ A Excitation depends more on the influx of extracellular calcium than release from internal stores

○ B It contains no actin or myosin filaments

○ C It classically relaxes when it is stretched

○ D It contains an extensive T-tubular system

○ E It is innervated through somatic motor nerve endings

77 ► With regard to the structure of cardiac muscle:

○ A The T-tubules are located at the junction of the A and I bands

○ B Cardiac muscle has no visible striations in their cytoplasm

○ C It has an underdeveloped sarcoplasmic reticulum

○ D There are specialised intercellular junctions between myocytes

○ E Muscle fibres are typically multinucleate with peripherally located nuclei

78

Cardiac muscle has which of the following properties?

○ A A fused tetanic response can be produced by repetitive stimulation

○ B The cardiac muscle action potential lasts approximately 2–3 ms

○ C Excitation–contraction coupling requires calcium-induced calcium release

○ D The force of contraction is independent of the length of the muscle fibre

○ E The plateau phase of the cardiac action potential is principally caused by sodium influx

79

With regard to the chemical neurotransmitters:

○ A Norepinephrine (noradrenaline) is the predominant neurotransmitter found between first- and second-order sympathetic neurons

○ B The nerve endings of second-order parasympathetic neurons release acetylcholine, which acts on nicotinic cholinergic receptors

○ C The neuromuscular junction releases acetylcholine, which acts on muscarinic cholinergic receptors

○ D The nucleus accumbens and substantia nigra are rich in dopamine

○ E The locus ceruleus and periaqueductal grey are rich in acetylcholine

Cardiovascular physiology
Questions

80 Cardiac output is decreased:

- ○ A During stimulation of sympathetic nerves to the heart
- ○ B On cutting the vagus nerves to the heart
- ○ C By increasing the end-diastolic volume of the heart
- ○ D As a consequence of decreased pressure in the carotid sinus
- ○ E On standing up

81 With regard to the relationship of the electrocardiogram to the cardiac cycle:

- ○ A The P wave results from atrial repolarisation
- ○ B The QRS complex is caused by ventricular repolarisation
- ○ C The Q–T interval gives a rough indication of the duration of ventricular systole
- ○ D The first heart sound occurs at the same time as the P wave
- ○ E The second heart sound occurs at the same time as the QRS complex

Answers on page 195

82 ▶ Flow through a vessel:

○ A Is inversely proportional to the pressure head of flow

○ B Is inversely proportional to the radius

○ C Is directly proportional to the length of the tube

○ D Is directly proportional to the viscosity of blood passing through it

○ E Is directly proportional to the fourth power of the radius

83 ▶ Which of the following substances is a vasodilator?

○ A Angiotensin II

○ B Nitric oxide

○ C Norepinephrine

○ D Vasopressin

○ E Thromboxane A_2

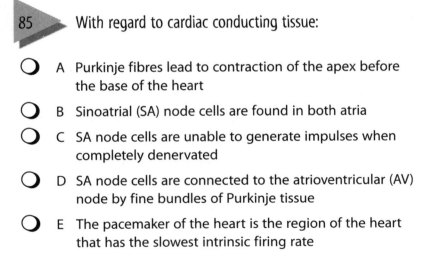

84 ▶ With regard to coronary blood flow (CBF):

○ A Blood flow to the left ventricle increases in early systole
○ B Local metabolic activity is the chief factor that determines the rate of blood flow to the heart
○ C CBF to the left ventricle increases in hypothermia
○ D CBF is increased in aortic stenosis
○ E The myocardium extracts 25% of the oxygen from the coronary blood

85 ▶ With regard to cardiac conducting tissue:

○ A Purkinje fibres lead to contraction of the apex before the base of the heart
○ B Sinoatrial (SA) node cells are found in both atria
○ C SA node cells are unable to generate impulses when completely denervated
○ D SA node cells are connected to the atrioventricular (AV) node by fine bundles of Purkinje tissue
○ E The pacemaker of the heart is the region of the heart that has the slowest intrinsic firing rate

Cardiovascular physiology – Questions

86 ▶ Circulating red blood cells (erythrocytes):

○ A Have a normal lifespan of 6–8 weeks

○ B Are broken down in the bone marrow

○ C Contain the enzyme glutaraldehyde anhydrase

○ D Lack nuclei and mitochondria

○ E Swell to bursting point when suspended in 0.9% saline

87 ▶ Erythrocytes:

○ A Travel at a slower velocity in venules than in capillaries

○ B Are normally spherical in shape

○ C Make little contribution to the buffering capacity of the blood

○ D After haemolysis release erythropoietin, which stimulates the production of more erythrocytes

○ E Deform as they pass through the capillaries

88 ▶ With regard to blood clotting:

○ A The haemostatic response comprises two key events

○ B Blood platelets have a small single-lobed nucleus

○ C The conversion of fibrinogen to fibrin is catalysed by prothrombin

○ D Blood clotting is reversed by plasmin (fibrinolysin)

○ E Liver failure results in a prothrombotic state

89 ▶ Which of the following is true with regard to the microcirculation and the formation of lymph?

○ A At the arterial end of the capillary, the plasma colloid osmotic pressure exceeds the capillary hydrostatic pressure

○ B At the venous end of the capillary, the capillary hydrostatic pressure exceeds the plasma colloid osmotic pressure

○ C Oedema results from a rise in colloid osmotic pressure

○ D Interstitial fluid hydrostatic pressure is normally negative

○ E All the fluid that is filtered from the capillary flows into lymph vessels

90 ▶ With regard to the cerebral circulation:

○ A Cerebral blood flow (CBF) is mainly governed by cardiovascular reflexes

○ B CBF is very sensitive to changes in the $P(co_2)$ of the perfusing blood

○ C CBF increases steeply with increasing blood pressure

○ D It comprises functional end arteries

○ E Raised intracranial pressure results in hypotension and tachycardia

Respiratory physiology
Questions

91 Which one of the following statements about lung volumes is true?

○ A The functional residual capacity is the sum of the tidal volume and residual volume

○ B The vital capacity is the sum of the inspiratory reserve volume, the expiratory reserve volume and the tidal volume

○ C The functional residual capacity can be measured directly by spirometry

○ D The residual volume is the volume of air left in the lungs after normal quiet expiration

○ E The normal tidal volume is about 2 litres

92 Surfactant:

○ A Increases the surface tension of the film of liquid lining the alveoli

○ B Reduces lung compliance

○ C Is secreted by type I pneumocytes

○ D Causes an increase in surface tension as the surface area of fluid decreases

○ E Helps to prevent the formation of pulmonary oedema

93 With regard to pulmonary blood flow:

○ A Dilatation of pulmonary blood vessels occurs in response to hypoxia

○ B The pulse pressure in the pulmonary artery is about the same as that in the aorta

○ C During exercise blood flow to the upper portion of the lung increases

○ D The ventilation–perfusion ratio is the same in all parts of the lung in a standing person

○ E Pulmonary vascular resistance is six times greater than that of the systemic circulation

▶ **94** With regard to chemoreceptors:

○ A The carotid bodies have a blood flow per unit volume similar to that of the brain

○ B The carotid bodies are stretch receptors in the walls of the carotid arteries

○ C Central chemoreceptors are located in the aortic arch

○ D Carotid bodies primarily respond to hypoxia

○ E The response of the peripheral chemoreceptors to arterial $Pa(co_2)$ is more important than that of the central chemoreceptors

▶ **95** Carbon dioxide transport:

○ A Carbon dioxide is mainly carried in the blood in its dissolved form

○ B CO_2 is carried as carboxyhaemoglobin on the haemoglobin molecule

○ C The Haldane effect describes changes in the affinity of the blood for CO_2 with variations in the $Pa(co_2)$

○ D Venous blood has a higher pH than arterial blood

○ E CO_2 is less soluble in plasma than O_2

96 ▶ The haemoglobin–oxygen dissociation curve:

○ A Is a rectangular hyperbola

○ B Is shifted to the left by an increase in $P(CO_2)$

○ C Is shifted to the right by fetal haemoglobin

○ D Demonstrates the Haldane effect, which describes the changes in affinity of the haemoglobin chain for O_2 after variations in the $Pa(CO_2)$

○ E Has a shape that is explained by the physicochemical properties of haemoglobin

97 ▶ At high altitude when the atmospheric pressure is halved, which one of the following changes occurs?

○ A Decreased pulmonary arterial pressure

○ B A decrease in arterial pH

○ C An increase in arterial $Pa(CO_2)$

○ D Decreased pulmonary ventilation

○ E An increase in blood viscosity

98 ▶ With regard to gas exchange:

○ A The rate of diffusion across the alveolar wall is directly proportional to its thickness

○ B Under resting conditions, equilibration between alveolar $P(o_2)$ and red blood cell $P(o_2)$ occurs one-third of the way along the pulmonary capillary

○ C At rest the red blood cell spends about 5 seconds within the pulmonary capillary

○ D The rate of diffusion across the alveolar wall is inversely proportional to the surface area available for diffusion

○ E Chlorine is the gas of choice for measuring the diffusion properties of the lung

99 ▶ With regard to the mechanics of respiration:

○ A Compliance is defined as the change in pressure per unit volume

○ B Compliance is synonymous with elastance

○ C Sighing serves no physiological purpose

○ D The lung follows the same behaviour in inflation and deflation

○ E Emphysema results in increased lung compliance

With regard to haemoglobin:

○ A Most of the haemoglobin circulates as free protein in plasma

○ B Oxygen attaches to the globin chains

○ C Each haemoglobin molecule combines with eight oxygen atoms

○ D In normal adult haemoglobin, iron exists in the ferric state

○ E Normal adult haemoglobin contains two α and two γ chains

Renal physiology
Questions

101 ▶ Erythropoietin:

○ A Is a polypeptide
○ B Has decreased secretion at high altitude
○ C In the adult is mainly made in the liver
○ D Acts via a secondary messenger
○ E Has its production decreased by local hypoxia

102 ▶ Which of the following is true with regard to aldosterone?

○ A Aldosterone is a steroid hormone secreted by the adrenal medulla
○ B Production is decreased by angiotensin-converting enzyme inhibitors
○ C Secretion results in increased potassium reabsorption from the nephron
○ D Secretion results in a rise in urinary pH
○ E Production ceases after the removal of the kidneys and their juxtaglomerular cells

With regard to the renin–angiotensin system:

○ A Angiotensinogen is secreted by the juxtaglomerular apparatus

○ B The lung catalyses the conversion of angiotensinogen to angiotensin I

○ C Activation results in the stimulation of aldosterone release

○ D Angiotensin II is a potent vasodilator

○ E Angiotensin-converting enzyme is principally found in the liver

With regard to the juxtaglomerular apparatus:

○ A The macula densa is a specialised region of the afferent arteriole

○ B Renin is secreted at the macula densa

○ C Renin is secreted in response to a raised sodium level at the macula densa

○ D A fall in pressure in the afferent arteriole promotes renin secretion

○ E The juxtaglomerular (granular) cells are located in the wall of the distal convoluted tubule

Antidiuretic hormone (ADH or arginine vasopressin):

○ A Increases in response to a ≥ 10% loss of circulating volume

○ B Is secreted by the pars distalis (adenohypophysis)

○ C Shows increased secretion in response to hypo-osmolar blood

○ D Causes water reabsorption from the loop of Henle

○ E When there is insufficiency, results in diabetes mellitus

With regard to acid–base balance:

○ A The normal pH of arterial blood is 7.85–7.95

○ B The pH of the blood fluctuates widely

○ C The kidneys respond fastest to a change in pH

○ D The kidney is able to generate new bicarbonate from glutamine

○ E The renal tubule reabsorbs hydrogen ions and actively excretes bicarbonate

107 ▶ With regard to renal blood flow:

○ A The kidneys receive 5% of the cardiac output

○ B Angiotensin II vasoconstricts the afferent more than the efferent arterioles

○ C Renal blood flow can be accurately measured by the use of inulin

○ D The low blood flow in the vasa recta assists in the formation of a concentrated urine

○ E A fall in arterial blood pressure decreases the glomerular filtration rate (GFR)

108 ▶ With regard to glomerular filtration:

○ A The GFR is the main factor determining the rate of urine production

○ B The GFR can be measured by the p-aminohippuric acid (PAH) concentration

○ C The normal GFR is 50 mL/min

○ D The glomerular filtration barrier comprises three layers

○ E A normal plasma creatinine implies normal renal function

109 ▶ With regard to tubular function:

○ A Of the filtered sodium 50% is reabsorbed in the distal convoluted tubule

○ B Most glucose is reabsorbed in the loop of Henle

○ C The ascending limb of the loop of Henle is permeable to water

○ D Drinking seawater is better than drinking nothing at all if lost at sea

○ E The maximum concentrating ability of the human kidney is 1200 mOsmol/L

Gastrointestinal physiology
Questions

110 With regard to saliva:

○ A Secretion is equivalent to 200 mL/day

○ B Secretion from the parotid gland is mainly mucinous

○ C It contains the trypsin enzyme

○ D It is richer in potassium than any other gastrointestinal secretion

○ E Secretion is a passive process

111 Which of the following cells secrete intrinsic factor?

○ A Goblet cells

○ B Kupffer cells

○ C Peptic cells

○ D Chief cells

○ E Parietal cells

112 ▶ Gastric acid secretion:

○ A Is inhibited by gastrin

○ B Is potentiated by histamine

○ C Starts only when food enters the stomach

○ D Is stimulated by the glossopharyngeal nerve

○ E Is stimulated by somatostatin

113 ▶ Gastrin:

○ A Is secreted in the body of the stomach

○ B Is stimulated by low pH

○ C Stimulates gastric acid production

○ D Inhibits gastric motility

○ E Causes the Zollinger–Ellison syndrome when there is decreased secretion

114 ▶ The exocrine pancreas:

○ A Secretes digestive juices with a pH of 4–5
○ B Develops from a single ventral pancreatic bud
○ C Shows inhibited secretion by cholecystokinin
○ D Has its main stimulation for secretion during the intestinal phase
○ E Produces secretin

115 ▶ Which of the following is true with regard to pancreatic enzymes?

○ A Trypsin is a powerful activator of other pancreatic proteolytic enzymes
○ B The pancreas secretes enterokinase (enteropeptidase)
○ C Chymotrypsinogen activates trypsinogen to form trypsin
○ D The pancreas secretes proteases in their activated form
○ E The pancreas normally contains a trypsin activator

116 ▸ With regard to the endocrine pancreas:

○ A It secretes hormones into a highly branched ductal system

○ B Glucagon is secreted from β-islet cells

○ C Islets of Langerhans make up only 2% of the volume of the gland

○ D Somatostatin is secreted from α-islet cells

○ E Glucagon stimulates glycogenesis

117 ▸ With regard to bile:

○ A Bile salts are derived from the waste products of haemoglobin

○ B Bile is actively concentrated in the gallbladder

○ C Thirty per cent is reabsorbed by the enterohepatic circulation

○ D Bile contains enzymes required for the digestion of fat

○ E Accumulation of bile salts is responsible for causing jaundice

118 ▶ With regard to intestinal absorption:

○ A A greater volume of water is absorbed from the colon than from the small intestine

○ B Gastric acid assists in the absorption of iron

○ C Glucose is absorbed by a potassium co-transport mechanism

○ D Vitamin B_{12} is absorbed from the duodenum

○ E Sodium is absorbed at a rate proportional to body needs

119 ▶ In the setting of starvation:

○ A Glycogen stores last for 2 weeks

○ B Glucose is the only metabolic fuel that can be used by neurons

○ C The brain uses free amino acids when glucose levels begin to fall

○ D Protein is spared until relatively late

○ E Death occurs at around 21 days

Endocrine physiology and thermoregulation
Questions

120 Which one of the following hormones is secreted by the anterior pituitary?

○ A Testosterone
○ B Oxytocin
○ C Thyroid-stimulating hormone (TSH)
○ D Corticotrophin-releasing protein (CRH)
○ E Anti diuretic hormone (ADH)

121 Which one of these statements about type 2 diabetes mellitus is true?

○ A Type 2 diabetes mellitus usually presents with weight loss

○ B Ketones are found

○ C Type 2 diabetes is associated with HLA-DR3/4

○ D Identical twins show 90% concordance

○ E Type 2 diabetes usually presents in the teens

122 In diabetes mellitus:

○ A A fasting glucose of 6.5 mmol/L is compatible with a diagnosis

○ B A random glucose of 9 mmol/L on two occasions is compatible with a diagnosis

○ C A fasting glucose of 7.5 mmol/L on two occasions is consistent with a diagnosis

○ D A glucose of 10 mmol/L after a 2-hour glucose tolerance test is compatible with a diagnosis

○ E A 50 g glucose challenge is used in the glucose tolerance test

123 Which of these statements about insulin is true?

○ A Insulin receptors use cAMP as their signal transducer
○ B Insulin is secreted by α cells in the pancreas
○ C Secretion is stimulated by somatostatin
○ D It is an anabolic hormone
○ E Insulin release is inhibited by the ingestion of amino acids

124 With regard to the hypothalamic–pituitary axis:

○ A Oxytocin is synthesised in the posterior pituitary gland
○ B Prolactin is under dominant inhibitory regulation
○ C Thyroxine is a steroid hormone
○ D Thyroid-stimulating hormone (TSH) acts via tyrosine kinase receptors
○ E Growth hormone (GH) binds to intracellular receptors

125 Cortisol:

○ A Is a protein
○ B Lowers blood glucose
○ C Is an anabolic hormone
○ D Is stimulated by renin
○ E Has a peak hormonal concentration in the morning

126 With regard to calcium homoeostasis:

○ A The active form of vitamin D is
25-hydroxycholecalciferol
○ B Parathyroid hormone (PTH) secretion is stimulated by
the pituitary gland
○ C Activated vitamin D decreases calcium absorption from
the intestine
○ D PTH acts directly on osteoblasts in bone
○ E In the kidney, PTH increases calcium excretion and
increases phosphate reabsorption from the urine

127 With regard to thyroxine (T_4):

○ A The thyroid gland produces more tri-iodothyronine or T_3 than T_4

○ B Thyroid hormone-releasing hormone (TRH) directly results in T_4 release from the thyroid gland

○ C T_4 promotes the growth and development of the brain

○ D T_4 decreases basal metabolic rate

○ E T_4 acts on cell surface receptors

128 During diabetic ketoacidosis:

○ A The pH of the blood is high

○ B Cheyne–Stokes breathing is characteristic

○ C Hyperkalaemia occurs

○ D Blood glucose levels are typically low

○ E The volume status is euvolaemic

With regard to adrenal gland disorders:

○ A Adrenal insufficiency results in hypokalaemia and hypernatraemia

○ B Conn syndrome results in hyperkalaemia

○ C Cushing's disease is the result of a cortisol-producing tumour of the adrenal cortex

○ D Phaeochromocytoma results from oversecretion of cortisol by a tumour of the adrenal medulla

○ E Congenital adrenal hyperplasia (adrenogenital syndrome) results in virilisation and salt wasting

130 Testosterone:

○ A Secretion occurs only in males

○ B Is secreted from the Sertoli cells of the testis

○ C Is a peptide hormone

○ D Is essential for spermatogenesis

○ E Depends on follicle-stimulating hormone (FSH) for secretion

131 ▶ Concerning the female reproductive system:

○ A The menopause is associated with an increase in FSH

○ B Oestrogen concentration peaks just before menstruation

○ C Both oestrogen and progesterone are necessary for ovulation to take place

○ D Oestrogen production is confined to ovarian tissue

○ E Fertilisation of the human ovum normally takes place in the uterus

132 ▶ Thermoregulation:

○ A Brown fat (non-shivering thermogenesis) plays a significant role in adults

○ B Acclimatisation of the sweating mechanism occurs in response to heat

○ C Apocrine sweat glands play an important role in heat loss by evaporation

○ D Thermoregulation is one of the principal functions of the thalamus

○ E Heat adaptation takes about 3–5 days to develop

Nerve, muscle and neuroscience

Answers

68 **C Upon exposure to light, cGMP levels within the photoreceptor fall**

Phototransduction is the process by which light energy in the form of photons is converted to a change in membrane potential of the photoreceptor cell (rod or cone).

Incident light photons
↓
Conformational change of rhodopsin
↓
Activation of G-protein, transducin
↓
Activation of cGMP phosphodiesterase
↓
Decreased intracellular cGMP
↓
Closure of Na⁺ channels
↓
Hyperpolarisation
↓
Decreased release of neurotransmitter
↓
Response in bipolar cells and other retinal neurons

Nerve, muscle and neuroscience – Answers

The outer segment of the rod contains internal membranous discs that contain the light-sensitive protein rhodopsin. Rhodopsin consists of opsin (seven transmembrane protein, or serpentine receptor) bound to retinal (the light-absorbing portion), a derivative of vitamin A. Deficiencies in vitamin A can therefore lead to night blindness and, if untreated, to deterioration of receptor outer segments and eventually total blindness. Slight differences among the opsins of each of the three types of cones result in differences in the wavelengths absorbed preferentially by each photopigment.

In the dark, non-selective cation channels in the outer segment are bound to cGMP and open, causing a predominant Na^+ influx. This is known as the dark current. The level of cGMP in the outer segment depends on its rate of synthesis (by guanylyl cyclase) and degradation (by phosphodiesterase). Absorption of a photon of light leads to isomerisation of retinal (from the 11-*cis* to the all-*trans* configuration), structural activation of rhodopsin and activation of the G-protein, transducin. Activated transducin produces a fall in cGMP, closure of cGMP-gated cation channels and hyperpolarisation. The hyperpolarisation reduces the release of synaptic transmitter (glutamate) and this generates a signal that ultimately leads to action potentials in ganglion cells (the output cells of the retina). The action potentials are transmitted to the brain. In a sense, therefore, our photoreceptors are really 'dark receptors', depolarising and releasing more transmitter as the level of illumination decreases. Presumably as we spend less than half our time in darkness this arrangement is not as metabolically inefficient as it at first sounds.

This seemingly cumbersome process occurs very rapidly and results in great amplification. Photoactivation of a single rhodopsin molecule can lead to the hydrolysis of more than 10^5 molecules of cGMP per second. The amplification helps to explain the remarkable sensitivity of photoreceptors; rods are capable of producing a detectable response to as little as one photon of light. Several forms of retinitis pigmentosa, an inherited disorder of photoreceptors leading to blindness, are caused by mutations within genes encoding members of the photoreceptor visual transduction cascade.

69 **D   The macular region is grossly over-represented in the visual cortex**

The visual pathway may be summarised as follows:

- Photoreceptors (rods, cones) within the retina convert light energy into electrical impulses (phototransduction).

- This is transmitted to ganglion cells, directly via bipolar cells or indirectly via horizontal and amacrine cells.

- Ganglion cells are the output cells of the retina. Axons from ganglion cells converge at the optic disc (blind spot) and travel in the optic nerve.

- Incomplete decussation occurs at the optic chiasma; those from the nasal half of each retina (corresponding to the temporal halves of the visual field) cross over (decussate) whereas those from the temporal halves of each retina stay on the same side.

- The optic tracts synapse in the various layers of the lateral geniculate nucleus of the thalamus before being relayed to the primary visual cortex in the occipital lobe via the optic radiation.

The macula is a region of the retina that subserves highest visual acuity. It is grossly over-represented in the visual cortex in a phenomenon known as cortical magnification. This may partly explain why lesions located within the visual cortex may result in macula sparing.

The effects of lesions to the visual pathway may be easily predicted using the above information:

- Lesions anterior to the optic chiasma (ie a transected optic nerve) result in a unilaterally blind eye.

- Lesions of the optic chiasma (commonly from a pituitary tumour) result in a bitemporal hemianopia.

- Lesions posterior to the optic chiasma (commonly as a result of ischaemic events) result in a homonymous hemianopia, with or without macula sparing.

70   B   The primary visual cortex is located within Broca's area

The human cerebral cortex is divided up into about 50 distinct areas known as the Brodmann areas based on histological structural differences. The numbered areas have come to refer to the different functional areas of the human cortex.

In general, sensory signals from all modalities of sensation terminate in the cerebral cortex posterior to the central sulcus (with the primary somatosensory cortex area lying in the postcentral gyrus). On the other hand, the portion of the cortex anterior to the central sulcus is devoted almost entirely to motor control (with the primary motor cortical area lying in the precentral gyrus). A good way to remember this is 'Marks and Spencer', or M&S, with motor in front and sensory behind the central sulcus.

Visual signals terminate in the occipital lobe (Brodmann area 17 corresponds to the primary visual cortex) and auditory signals terminate in the temporal lobe (Heschl's gyrus).

There are two primary language centres within the brain – Broca's and Wernicke's areas. Broca's area is situated in the frontoparietal area and is concerned with the expression of speech. Wernicke's area lies in the temporoparietal area and deals primarily with the comprehension of speech. In most people, the left cerebral hemisphere is dominant so that a stroke affecting the left cerebral cortex (resulting in a right-sided hemiparesis) wipes out the language centres, producing a corresponding dysphasia.

71 ▶ E Turns over approximately four to five times daily

Cerebrospinal fluid (CSF), situated within the ventricles and the subarachnoid space, bathes the surface of the brain and spinal cord, supplies nutrients to it, protects it and reduces its effective buoyancy. It also plays an important homoeostatic role and is crucial for maintaining a constant external environment for neurons and glia. In humans the volume is about 150 mL and its rate of production is 0.5 mL/min (or about 30 mL/h or 600 mL/day). Thus, the CSF turns over about four times daily.

Most of the CSF is produced by the choroid plexus, which is situated in the lateral, third and fourth ventricles. It flows between the lateral ventricles and third ventricle via the interventricular foramen (of Monro). The third and fourth ventricles communicate via the cerebral aqueduct (or aqueduct of Sylvius). The fourth ventricle communicates with the spinal cord by way of the single median foramen of Magendie and the two laterally placed foramina of Luschka. CSF is absorbed directly into the cerebral venous sinuses through the arachnoid villi, or granulations, by a process known as mass or bulk flow.

Occasionally the above physiology is disrupted and it becomes the centre of a pathological process. Hydrocephalus is an increase in the volume of CSF within the cerebral ventricles. It may arise from the oversecretion of CSF, impaired absorption of CSF or obstruction of CSF pathways.

C   The protein content of the CSF is 0.5% that of plasma

The constituents of the CSF are regulated by an active process that takes place within the choroid plexus. Thus, the composition of the CSF differs from that of plasma. Of importance are the concentrations of K^+, Ca^{2+}, bicarbonate and protein, which are lower in the CSF than in the plasma. This is to prevent high concentrations of these electrolytes inadvertently exciting neurons present within the brain substance.

The potassium content of the CSF is particularly important in this respect. Further buffering of the K^+ content of CSF take place through astrocytes.

Likewise, the low protein content of the CSF (the CSF protein content is 0.5% that of plasma) is deliberate to prevent some proteins and amino acids acting as 'false neurotransmitters'. The CSF is more acidic than plasma because its pH plays a critical role in the regulation of pulmonary ventilation and cerebral blood flow. Another reason why the CSF protein is kept deliberately low is to prevent proteins buffering the pH. The result is that the pH of the CSF accurately reflects CO_2 levels in the blood. In this way changes in pH act as a powerful regulator of the respiratory system (through the action of pH on central chemoreceptors) and act on cerebral blood flow.

73 ▶ B Increasing membrane capacitance

The speed of nerve conduction increases with:

- increasing axonal diameter, which decreases axonal resistance
- myelination (insulation of axons) by Schwann cells in the peripheral nervous system, or oligodendrocytes in the central nervous system (CNS)
- increasing temperature
- decreasing membrane capacitance.

Capacitance slows down passive conduction because some of the current has to be used to charge or discharge the capacitance before it can spread further.

The effect of temperature on axonal velocity is easily understood by remembering what happens to our hands when playing in the snow on a cold day. Most of us will be able to recall that our hands go numb, but retain the ability to feel pain. The reason is straightforward and is based on axonal velocity. Light touch is carried by myelinated Aβ nerve fibres. As the temperature decreases, the velocity of impulse propagation decreases until a point comes at which the amplitude of impulse is insufficient to regenerate the action potential at the next node of Ranvier. Cooling has the further effect of slowing sodium conductance at the nodes of Ranvier. Saltatory conduction is therefore disrupted, the result being that the hands are numb. Pain, on the other hand, is carried by unmyelinated C fibres. The generation of action potentials is not therefore restricted to the nodes of Ranvier and pain sensation is preserved until far lower temperatures are reached.

The myelin sheath increases velocity by three mechanisms: first, by insulating the axon; second, by decreasing membrane capacitance; and, third, by restricting the generation of axon potentials to the nodes of Ranvier. The importance of myelination in increasing the speed of nerve conduction is illustrated by certain disease states where the myelin sheath is absent or lacking. One example is the condition multiple sclerosis, which is a chronic, inflammatory, demyelinating condition that results in multifocal lesions within the white matter of the CNS. The equivalent disease process within the peripheral nervous system is known as Guillain–Barré syndrome. Both result in neurological deficits, such as motor weakness and sensory loss as a result of the decreased velocity of impulse propagation down nerve fibres.

74 ▶ E Contains intracellular stores of calcium ions

A single motor neuron supplies a group of muscle fibres in what is known as a motor unit. The more precise the movement, the fewer the muscle fibres supplied by one motor neuron. However, each muscle fibre is innervated by only one motor neuron.

Mammalian skeletal muscle is optimally organised for rapid excitation of muscle contraction in a process known as excitation–contraction coupling. Calcium is released from the intracellular stores (sarcotubular system) when skeletal muscle contracts. Calcium reuptake occurs through an active mechanism that needs a calcium pump. During contraction the actin and myosin filaments do not shorten but slide together over each other (sliding filament theory).

Decreasing extracellular calcium increases excitability and may lead to spontaneous contractions (tetany), possibly by increasing sodium permeability. In hypocalcaemia this may manifest clinically as Chvostek's sign (activation of the facial nerve and muscles by merely tapping the skin) or Trousseau's sign (carpopedal spasm producing the 'main d'accoucheur'). Fatal spasm of the larynx and seizures may later ensue if calcium levels are not corrected. Hyperventilation (overbreathing) may cause a similar effect through the respiratory alkalosis that it generates. Amino acids buffer the change in pH by losing protons to the plasma; in doing so, they become negatively charged. This negative charge binds free calcium in the plasma, resulting in hypocalcaemia.

75   **D   The equilibrium potential for an ion species depends on the ratio of the concentrations of the ion outside and inside the cell**

In axons, impulses can travel in both directions (orthodromic and antidromic) from a point of electrical stimulation. Antidromic activity explains certain clinical phenomena such as how infection of a dorsal root by herpes zoster virus causes the segmental cutaneous hyperaemia characteristic of 'shingles'.

The amplitude of the action potential generated by an excitatory stimulus is independent of the stimulus strength. This is known as the 'all or nothing' law, which means that stimulus intensity is coded for by frequency rather than through the amplitude of action potential.

The resting membrane potential is dependent on the electrogenic Na^+/K^+ ATPase pump and the relative intracellular and extracellular concentrations of ions on either side of the nerve cell membrane, as well as their relative permeabilities across the membrane. This establishes both a concentration (chemical) gradient and an electrical gradient across the nerve cell membrane, ie an electrochemical gradient. The equilibrium potential for a given ion species depends on the ratio of the concentrations of the ion outside the cell to that inside (Nernst's potential or equation). The Goldman constant field (or Goldman–

Hodgkin–Katz) equation is a more general form of Nernst's equation that allows for different permeabilities. Resting nerve cell membranes are about 100 times more permeable to K^+ ions than to Na^+ ions.

If extracellular sodium is replaced by potassium it would follow from Nernst's equation that this would depolarise the fibres completely. The resulting depolarisation inactivates sodium channels and blocks the propagation of impulses down nerves. This is why hyperkalaemia is so dangerous. Cardiac muscle is especially sensitive to small changes in extracellular K^+ concentrations and death often ensues from cardiac standstill.

 76   A   Excitation depends more on the influx of extracellular calcium than release from internal stores

In smooth muscle actin and myosin filaments occur, but are less obvious on microscopy, giving it a non-striated appearance. Most smooth muscle has extensive electrically conducting gap junctions between cells, which allows propagation of waves of electrical excitation through the tissue.

Smooth muscle is usually under autonomic (involuntary nervous) or hormonal control, unlike skeletal muscle which is under somatic control. Unlike skeletal muscle, smooth muscle can generate active tension in the absence of any neural activity (latch bridge mechanism).

There is a vesicular sarcoplasmic reticulum close to the membrane (caveolae), but no T-tubular system. This is because the slow speed of smooth muscle does not require an elaborate mechanism for intracellular calcium release. For this reason and as a result of the higher surface area to volume ratio of smooth muscle cells, excitation depends more on the influx of extracellular calcium than release from internal stores, because smooth muscle has a less well-developed sarcoplasmic reticulum.

The intrinsic myogenic response in smooth muscle opposes stretch. The result is that contraction may be generated by mechanical stretch of muscle fibres, eg in blood vessel walls. This is partly the basis for autoregulation of blood flow in the cerebral, coronary and renal vascular beds. It also plays a role in the peristaltic movements of material in the intestine.

77   D There are specialised intercellular junctions between myocytes

The structure of cardiac muscle correlates beautifully with its function.

Certain features concerning cardiac myocytes are worth remembering:

- Cardiac myocytes are shorter than skeletal muscle cells.

- They are branched.

- Typically they contain a single, centrally placed nucleus (unlike skeletal muscle fibres that are multinucleate, with peripherally located nuclei).

- Intercalated discs with gap junctions result in a syncytium where adjacent cardiac cells are mechanically and electrically coupled to each other, optimising cardiac contractility.

- They are rich in mitochondria.

- They contain sarcoplasmic reticulum.

- Transverse tubules located at the Z-line. Note that in skeletal muscle the T-tubules are located at the junction of the A and I bands.

- The pacemaker cells have unstable resting membrane potentials.

- Cardiac muscle contracts spontaneously (myogenic).

- A property shared by skeletal and cardiac muscle is their striated microscopic appearance from the highly organised arrangement of actin and myosin filaments.

78   C   Excitation-contraction coupling requires calcuim-induced calcium release

The most important source of activator calcium in cardiac muscle remains its release from the sarcoplasmic reticulum, although calcium also enters from the extracellular space during the plateau phase of the action potential. This calcium entry provides the stimulus that induces calcium release from the sarcoplasmic reticulum (calcium-induced calcium release).

The result is that tension generated in cardiac, but not skeletal, muscle is profoundly influenced by both extracellular calcium levels and factors that affect the magnitude of the inward calcium current. This is of practical value in two key clinical situations: in heart failure where digoxin is used to increase cardiac contractility (by increasing the intracellular calcium concentration) and in hyperkalaemia where calcium gluconate is used to stabilise the myocardium.

The force of contraction of cardiac muscle is heavily dependent upon its stretched fibre length. This is the basis of the Frank–Starling mechanism, which adjusts the energy of cardiac contraction in response to diastolic stretch (filling). This autoregulatory mechanism makes the heart a self-regulating pump with respect to both demands from the peripheral circulation and the balance of the pumping by the right and left sides of the heart.

The plateau phase of the action potential in cardiac muscle (principally resulting from calcium influx) maintains the membrane at a depolarised potential for as long as 500 ms. The result is that the cell membrane is refractory throughout most of the mechanical response, largely as a result of the inactivation of fast sodium channels. This prevents tetany upon repetitive stimulation, which would be detrimental to cardiac output. Furthermore, the prolonged refractory period in cardiac muscle allows the impulse that originates in the sinoatrial node to propagate throughout the entire myocardium just once, thereby preventing re-entry arrhythmias.

79   D   The nucleus accumbens and substantia nigra are rich in dopamine

The nervous system can be arbitrarily divided into the somatic (or 'voluntary') and autonomic (or 'involuntary') nervous system. The autonomic nervous system consists of two arms, namely the sympathetic and parasympathetic nervous systems.

Both sympathetic and parasympathetic fibres consist of two neurons (first-order, or preganglionic, and second-order, or postganglionic, neurons) and two synapses (the synaptic cleft between the first- and second-order neurons and the synaptic cleft between the second-order neuron and the organ or effector). There are key differences between both the neurons and the synapses of the sympathetic and parasympathetic nervous systems.

First-order (preganglionic) sympathetic and parasympathetic neurons are myelinated, whereas second-order (postganglionic) sympathetic and parasympathetic neurons are small, unmyelinated fibres. In both the sympathetic and parasympathetic nervous systems, preganglionic neurons release acetylcholine, which acts on postsynaptic nicotinic cholinergic receptors. However, they differ at the second synapse (between second-order neurons and the effector) where norepinephrine is the principal chemical neurotransmitter used within the sympathetic nervous system (although this is not entirely true because the postganglionic sympathetic nerve fibres to the sweat glands, the piloerector muscles and a few blood vessels are cholinergic), but acetylcholine is the principal neurotransmitter used within the parasympathetic nervous system (although this time acting on muscarinic cholinergic receptors).

The neuromuscular junction (the synapse between somatic motor neurons and skeletal muscle) operates via acetylcholine acting through nicotinic acetylcholine receptors. The substantia nigra is a dense area of dopaminergic neurons that forms part of the basal ganglia; degeneration leads to Parkinson's disease. The periaqueductal grey is a region rich in endogenous opioids, which are believed to play a pivotal role in attenuation of painful stimuli through descending inhibition from higher centres. The noradrenergic receptor-rich locus ceruleus is believed to play a key role in attention. The nucleus accumbens is dopamine rich and plays an important role in addiction and reward. The adrenal medulla is an endocrine gland, but is effectively a specialised second-order (postganglionic) sympathetic nerve terminal that secretes approximately 70% epinephrine and 30% norepinephrine. Excess catecholamines are secreted by the adrenal medulla in a condition known as a phaeochromocytoma, which is a rare tumour of the adrenal gland. A thorough grounding of the aforementioned chemical neurotransmitters is imperative if we are to understand certain disease states and how particular drugs act within the nervous system.

Cardiovascular physiology
Answers

 80   E   On standing up

There are two key equations worth remembering relating to cardiovascular physiology:

$$CO = HR \times SV$$

where CO is cardiac output, HR is heart rate and SV is stroke volume.

$$MABP = CO \times TPR$$

where MABP is mean arterial blood pressure, CO is cardiac output and TPR is total peripheral resistance.

Stimulation of the sympathetic nervous system results in a rise in heart rate and stroke volume and therefore cardiac output increases. Cutting the vagus nerves to the heart results in an increase in heart rate because of the abolition of vagal tone, so cardiac output increases.

If the end-diastolic volume of the heart (preload) is increased, under normal physiological circumstances, cardiac output is increased by the Frank–Starling–Sarnoff mechanism. The exception is in the failing heart where the law of LaPlace becomes more important and cardiac output actually falls.

Arterial blood pressure is homoeostatically regulated through the action of baroreceptors, which are principally located in the carotid sinus and the wall of the aortic arch. If the carotid sinus pressure is reduced, the baroreceptors become inactive and lose their inhibitory effect on the vasomotor centre in the brain stem. The vasomotor centre then becomes much more active, resulting in activation of the sympathetic nervous system. This produces a rise in heart rate, stroke volume, mean systemic filling pressure and venous return, causing an increase in cardiac output and return of the mean arterial blood pressure to its original value.

Cardiac output drops when we stand up as a result of the pooling of blood on the venous side of the circulation, which has a large capacitance. Stepping out of a hot bath exacerbates this pooling effect because superficial cutaneous veins dilate in response to heat, which increases their capacitance even further. Under normal physiological circumstances, activation of the baroreceptor reflex compensates to some degree, preventing fainting (syncope). However, in elderly people, or patients on blood pressure-lowering drugs, inadequate compensation from the baroreceptor reflex may result in a vasovogal syncope or orthostatic hypotension.

81   C   The Q-T interval gives a rough indication of the duration of ventricular systole

It is important to understand the nature of the electrocardiogram (ECG). As a junior doctor you will read and interpret ECGs every day at work:

P wave = atrial depolarisation

QRS complex = ventricular depolarisation

T wave = ventricular repolarisation.

(Electrical activity resulting from atrial repolarisation is 'hidden' within the QRS complex.)

The Q–T interval gives a rough indication of the duration of ventricular systole. The first heart sound results from closure of the AV valves and occurs as the ventricles contract. It therefore coincides with the QRS complex. The second heart sound is caused by closure of the aortic and pulmonary valves, respectively, and occurs at about the same time as the T wave.

82   E   Is directly proportional to the fourth power of the radius

The Hagen–Poiseuille law states that the flow through a vessel is:

- directly proportional to the pressure head of flow
- directly proportional to the fourth power of radius
- inversely proportional to the viscosity
- inversely proportional to the length of the tube.

The radius of the tube is therefore the most important determinant of flow through a blood vessel, and doubling the radius of the tube will lead to a 16-fold increase in flow at a constant pressure gradient. The implications of this are severalfold.

First, owing to the fourth power effect on resistance and flow, active changes in radius constitute an extremely powerful mechanism for regulating both the local blood flow to a tissue and central arterial pressure. The arterioles are the main resistance vessels of the circulation and their radius can be actively controlled by the tension of smooth muscle within its wall.

Second, in terms of intravenous fluid replacement in hospital, flow is greater through a peripheral cannula than through central lines. The reason is that peripheral lines are short and wide (and therefore of lower resistance and higher flow) compared with central lines, which are long and possess a narrow lumen. A peripheral line is therefore preferential to a central line when urgent fluid resuscitation, or blood, is required.

▶ B   Nitric oxide

The importance of endothelium in vascular responses was first noted when it was discovered that removing the endothelium from perfused arteries prevented the vasodilator action of acetylcholine on those vessels. The endothelium-derived relaxing factor has since been recognised as nitric oxide (a vasodilator). Vasopressin, angiotensin II, thromboxane A_2 and norepinephrine are all vasoconstrictors.

Since its discovery, nitric oxide has been implicated in a diverse array of different biological processes, both physiological and pathological, besides vasodilatation, including:

- acting as a neurotransmitter
- the killing of micro-organisms by phagocytes
- long-term potentiation (memory)
- male erection (note that Viagra [sildenafil] enhances the effect of nitric oxide)
- sepsis
- excitotoxicity.

In addition nitric oxide explains how glyceryl trinitrate exerts its beneficial effect in angina. More is being discovered about nitric oxide all the time.

84 B Local metabolic activity is the chief factor that determines the rate of blood flow to the heart

Given that there is a high myocardial oxygen demand at rest (around 20 times that of skeletal muscle), certain functional adaptations ensure that supply adequately meets demand:

- The heart receives 4–5% of the cardiac output.

- High capillary density.

- High oxygen extraction ratio – the myocardium extracts around 70% of the oxygen that is delivered to it from the coronary blood; in contrast, the body average is only 25%.

- Efficient metabolic hyperaemia, where local metabolism is the dominant controller of coronary flow – the extra oxygen required at high work rates is supplied chiefly by an increase in blood flow rather than an increase in the oxygen extraction ratio.

Unlike other vascular beds, the coronary flow to the left ventricle is greatest in diastole. This occurs as a result of the mechanical compression of the coronary vessels during systole, such that there is reversal of the transmural pressure gradient across the vessel wall, leading to momentary occlusion. Coronary perfusion is reduced in aortic stenosis (narrowing) because the coronary ostia lie distal to the aortic valve. This is why patients with aortic stenosis get angina.

In hypothermia there is a fall in metabolic rate and cardiac output. This reduces cardiac work, resulting in a decrease in the rate of production of vasodilator metabolites (such as adenosine, CO_2). The reduction in coronary artery perfusion pressure explains why angina is commonly triggered by exposure to the cold.

A   Purkinje fibres lead to contraction of the apex before the base of the heart

The group of cells that show the highest automaticity (ie the cells with which the resting membrane potential drifts towards the threshold fastest) dictates the overall heart rate and is accordingly called the primary intrinsic pacemaker of the heart. These are normally the pacemaker cells from the SA node, which discharge at about 60–80 times every minute.

The SA node is found in the right atrium near its junction with the superior vena cava. The SA node receives a rich innervation from both arms of the autonomic nervous system (sympathetic and parasympathetic). By this means they can exert a powerful extrinsic influence on the heart.

Atrial fibres conduct impulses from the SA node to the AV node. The latter provides the only communication in the normal heart between the atria and ventricles. Conduction through the AV node is slower than through the remaining myocardium; this synchronises the sequential atrial and ventricular contraction. Purkinje fibres are confined to the ventricles.

Impulse generation is a result of spontaneous diastolic depolarisation of the cells. The SA node has intrinsic rhythmicity and can generate impulses independently, even when completely denervated.

Purkinje fibres are larger than ventricular myocardial cells and this facilitates the rapid spread of depolarisation over the entire ventricular myocardium. Purkinje fibres travel to the apex before proceeding to the base of the heart. This arrangement enables the activation wave to spread from the apex to the base of the ventricles. The resulting pattern of activation leads to a ventricular contraction from apex to base, which optimises the extrusion of blood from the chambers.

Problems with cardiac conduction are commonly encountered in clinical practice. Arrhythmias are the most common cause of death after a myocardial infarction. In the event that the SA node function is abnormal, as in sick sinus syndrome, or after myocardial ischaemia, other sites with a slower intrinsic rate can substitute the role of the pacemaker, resulting in an escape rhythm.

86 ▶ D Lack nuclei and mitochondria

Erythrocytes do not contain nuclei (they are anucleate) or mitochondria. This maximises the haemoglobin-carrying capacity of red cells. The absence of mitochondria precludes aerobic energy production; hence they are very efficient O_2 transporters because they do not consume any O_2 directly.

Erythrocytes are thus totally dependent on the anaerobic metabolism of glucose to generate the energy needed to maintain electrochemical gradients across their cell membranes.

Without nuclei, erythrocytes are unable to replace deteriorating enzymes and membrane proteins; this shortens their life expectancy. The average lifespan of a normal erythrocyte is 120 days (or 16–18 weeks). Lifespan may be reduced further as a result of the premature destruction of red cells. This is a feature of haemolysis. Aged red cells are removed from the circulation by the spleen and liver.

Erythrocytes contain the enzyme carbonic anhydrase, which catalyses the reaction $CO_2 + H_2O = H^+ + HCO_3^-$ and requires zinc as a co-factor. This plays an important role in CO_2 transport and the buffering of pH.

Erythrocytes do not burst when placed in 0.9% (physiological or normal) saline because this is isotonic with their contents.

Unstressed erythrocytes normally appear as biconcave discs. This provides a 20–30% greater surface area than a sphere relative to cell volume, thus significantly enhancing gaseous exchange. This shape, with the fluidity of the plasma membrane, allows the erythrocyte to deform easily, thus making erythrocytes able to pass through the smallest capillaries. They appear spherical in a genetic condition known as hereditary spherocytosis.

Normal red blood cells are around 7 μm in diameter, whereas the diameter of capillaries is only around 5 μm. Red cells possess deformable walls and therefore become bullet shaped as they pass through capillaries. This enables 'bolus flow' or 'plug flow', which eliminates some of the internal friction associated with laminae sliding over each other (Fahraeus–Lindqvist effect). The reduction in apparent viscosity means that capillaries have a lower resistance to flow than if blood were a uniform fluid containing the same amounts of protein, but without the red cell membrane to parcel it up. The efficiency of bolus flow depends critically on the deformability of the red cell and this deformability is impaired in many clinical conditions, the most dramatic of which is sickle cell anaemia.

Erythrocytes make a major contribution to the buffering capacity of the blood through the action of carbonic anhydrase and haemoglobin contained within the red cells. Indeed red cells are responsible for most of the buffering power of whole blood.

Erythropoiesis (the production of red cells) is stimulated by the hormone erythropoietin, although the main source of erythropoietin is the kidney, not the erythrocytes.

The capillary bed has a greater cross-sectional area than the venular bed. Blood therefore travels more slowly in capillaries compared with venules. This fact prolongs the time available for gaseous exchange. Red cells are not evenly distributed across the bloodstream in large blood vessels, but form an axial stream away from the vessel wall, leaving a cell-deficient layer of plasma at the margins. This marginal layer helps to ease the blood along.

88 D Blood clotting is reversed by plasmin (fibrinolysin)

One of the drawbacks of having a high-pressure circulation is that even slight damage to blood vessels, especially on the arterial side, can lead to a rapid loss of circulatory blood volume. To prevent bleeding we have developed quite complicated responses to vessel damage designed to stop bleeding.

Three key physiological events occur with the onset of bleeding:

1. Vasoconstriction

2. Platelet aggregation to form the primary haemostatic plug

3. Activation of the clotting cascade to form a fibrin plug (secondary or stable haemostatic plug).

The balance of all components – vessel wall, platelets, adhesive and coagulation proteins, and regulatory mechanisms – determines the effectiveness of the haemostatic plug in maintaining the structural and functional integrity of the circulatory system.

Blood platelets are formed from megakaryocytes in the bone marrow. They are anucleate, but the cytoplasm contains electron-dense granules, lysosomes and mitchondria. Each megakaryocyte is responsible for the production of around 4000 platelets. The half-life of platelets in the blood is about 8–12 days.

The clotting cascade involves a series of several highly specific serine proteases, which activate each other in a stepwise manner.

In this way, a rapid response is achieved because at each step the signal is amplified. Clotting factors are produced in the liver so that liver failure results in a tendency to bleed (anticoagulant state). The final stage of the clotting cascade involves the conversion of fibrinogen to fibrin; this is catalysed by thrombin, not prothrombin, which is the inactive precursor of thrombin.

Plasmin acts as a regulatory mechanism to keep the clotting cascade in check and to prevent the over-clotting of blood, which could have disastrous consequences (such as the occlusion of blood vessels). It degrades both fibrin and fibrinogen to products that can inhibit thrombin. Fibrinolytic agents are widely used in clinical practice – a good example being the use of thrombolytics in acute myocardial infarction.

89   D   Interstitial fluid hydrostatic pressure is normally negative

Four primary forces determine the movement of fluid across the capillary membrane (Starling's forces):

1. The capillary hydrostatic pressure – 'forces fluid out'.
2. The plasma colloid osmotic pressure – 'pulls fluid in'.
3. The interstitial fluid hydrostatic pressure – 'pushes fluid in'.
4. The interstitial fluid colloid osmotic pressure – 'pulls fluid out'.

At the arterial end of the capillary, the capillary hydrostatic pressure exceeds the plasma colloid osmotic pressure and fluid is drawn out of the capillary into the interstitium. By this means, transport of nutrients to the tissues occurs. However, as one moves along the capillary, the capillary hydrostatic pressure falls such that, at the venous end of the capillary, the plasma colloid osmotic pressure exceeds the capillary hydrostatic pressure and fluid moves back into the capillary, removing cellular excreta. In this way, about 90% of the fluid that has filtered out of the arterial ends of capillaries is reabsorbed at the venous ends. Only the remainder flows into the lymph vessels.

Interstitial fluid hydrostatic pressure is normally subatmospheric (negative). This results from the suction effect of the lymphatics returning fluid to the circulation, which maintains the structural integrity of the tissues, keeps the interstitial spaces small and reduces distances for diffusion.

Movement of lymph in one direction along the lymphatics depends on:

- Filtration pressure from capillaries
- Action of local muscles
- Action of local arterial pulsation
- Respiratory movement (thoracoabdominal pump) with intermittent negative pressures in the brachiocephalic veins
- Smooth muscle in the walls of larger lymphatics (sympathetically controlled)
- Valves within.

Oedema (excess fluid accumulation in the extracellular spaces) results from:

- Elevated capillary pressure
- Decreased plasma colloid osmotic pressure
- Increased interstitial fluid protein
- Increased capillary permeability
- Blockage of lymph return (lymphoedema).

Diffusion distances are greatly increased as a result of oedema and this can interfere with cell nutrition.

B **CBF is very sensitive to changes in the P(Co$_2$) of the perfusing blood**

The cerebral circulation does not consist of functional end-arteries. Rather, a rich vascular anastomosis known as the circle of Willis surrounds the base of the brain, into which all the main arteries to the brain connect so that, if one artery should block, the brain can still be supplied by the other arteries in this anastomotic arrangement.

Cerebral blood flow (CBF) is hardly affected by cardiovascular reflexes (ie the autonomic nervous system). CO_2 is the most important determinant of CBF, via its local vasodilator action (in under-perfused areas CO_2 accumulates and this leads to vasodilatation and restoration of normal cerebral perfusion). Hyperventilation leads to washout of CO_2 from the blood and constriction of cerebral blood vessels. This may result in syncope after a panic attack. In addition, it explains why hyperventilating before diving into water can result in syncope under water and drowning. The local effect of CO_2 on the cerebral vasculature is deliberately used in the management of head injury where hyperventilation is used to reduce raised intracranial pressure.

The rate of CBF remains essentially stable, up to a point, with changing blood pressure owing to local autoregulation of flow. Autoregulation is very well developed in the brain; a fall in blood pressure causes the resistance vessels to dilate and thereby maintain flow. Cerebral autoregulation seems to involve both myogenic and metabolic mechanisms.

The important interrelationship of cerebral perfusion, mean arterial blood pressure and intracranial pressure is as follows:

$$CPP = MABP - ICP$$

where CPP = cerebral perfusion pressure, MABP = mean arterial blood pressure and ICP = intracranial pressure.

It stems from the fact that the adult brain is enclosed in a rigid, incompressible box, with the result that the volume inside it must remain constant (Monroe–Kelly doctrine). A rise in intracranial pressure therefore decreases cerebral perfusion pressure (and hence CBF). In raised intracranial pressure, as the brain stem becomes compressed, local neuronal activity causes a rise in sympathetic vasomotor drive and thus a rise in blood pressure. This is known as Cushing's reflex. This elevated blood pressure evokes a bradycardia via the baroreceptor reflex. Cushing's reflex helps to maintain CBF and protect the vital centres of the brain from loss of nutrition if the intracranial pressure rises high enough to compress the cerebral arteries.

Respiratory physiology

Answers

 91 **B** The vital capacity is the sum of the inspiratory reserve volume, the expiratory reserve volume and the tidal volume

Spirometry traces are easy to understand if you remember the following two rules:

1. There are four lung volumes and five capacities that you need to remember.

2. A capacity is made up of two or more lung volumes.

The four lung volumes are:

1. Tidal volume = volume of air inspired or expired with each normal breath in quiet breathing – approximately 500 mL.

2. Residual volume = that volume of air remaining in the lung after forced expiration.

3. Inspiratory reserve volume = extra volume of air that can be inspired over and above the normal tidal volume.

4. Expiratory reserve volume = extra volume of air that can be expired by forceful expiration after the end of a normal tidal expiration.

The five lung capacities are:

1. Functional residual capacity (FRC) = that volume of air that remains in the lung at the end of quiet expiration. It is equal to the sum of the residual volume (RV) and the expiratory reserve volume.

2. Inspiratory capacity = inspiratory reserve volume + tidal volume

3. Expiratory capacity = expiratory reserve volume + tidal volume

4. Vital capacity = inspiratory reserve volume + tidal volume + expiratory reserve volume (or total lung capacity − RV)

5. Total lung capacity (TLC) = vital capacity + RV

The RV (and therefore FRC and TLC) cannot be measured directly by spirometry. They are measured by either whole body plethysmography or using the helium dilution or nitrogen washout techniques.

Surfactant is formed in and secreted by type II pneumocytes. The active ingredient is dipalmitoyl phosphatidylcholine, which helps prevent alveolar collapse by lowering the surface tension between water molecules in the surface layer. In this way it helps to reduce the work of breathing (makes the lungs more compliant) and permits the lung to be more easily inflated.

As the surfactant remains at the water–air interface, the space between surfactant molecules decreases as the surface area is reduced; this is equivalent to raising its concentration, which in turn lowers surface tension. This prevents alveolar collapse. Likewise, the decreasing effect of surfactant as the lungs inflate helps to prevent overinflation. This unique property of surfactant helps to stabilise different sizes of alveoli (otherwise the smaller alveoli would empty into the larger alveoli by LaPlace's law).

Surfactant is not produced in any significant quantity until week 32 of gestation and it then builds up to a high concentration by week 35 (the normal gestation period is 39 weeks). Premature delivery may therefore result in inadequate surfactant production and respiratory distress syndrome of the newborn (hyaline membrane disease).

Surfactant also plays an important role in keeping the alveoli dry. Just as the surface tension forces tend to collapse alveoli, they also tend to suck fluid into the alveolar spaces from the capillaries. By reducing these surface forces, surfactant prevents the transudation of fluid. In this way it acts as an important safety mechanism against the formation of pulmonary oedema.

ANSWERS

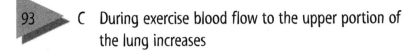

93   C   During exercise blood flow to the upper portion of the lung increases

Systolic and diastolic pressures in the pulmonary artery are about a sixth of those in the aorta and so is the pulse pressure. This is because the pulmonary vascular resistance is about a sixth of the systemic vascular resistance. The blood flow is the same in both circulations, otherwise blood would accumulate in one or other bed.

In a standing individual, blood flow is less in the upper parts of the lung than in the lower regions, but this is not matched by the differences in ventilation, so the ventilation–perfusion ratio is not the same in all parts of the lung. A standing individual has a higher ventilation–perfusion ratio at the apex than at the base.

During exercise, recruitment of the apical vessels accommodates the increase in cardiac output and pulmonary blood flow that occurs with exercise. This has the effect of increasing the area of capillaries available for gas exchange.

The pulmonary vasculature exhibits a peculiar property found nowhere else in the circulation, known as hypoxic pulmonary vasoconstriction. It consists of contraction of smooth muscle in the walls of the small arterioles in response to hypoxia – the opposite effect to that normally observed in the systemic circulation. The mechanism remains obscure. It has the effect of directing blood flow away from hypoxic regions of the lung (eg poorly ventilated areas of the diseased lung in adults) and in this way helps to optimise the local ventilation–perfusion ratios.

ANSWERS

MCQs in Applied Basic Sciences for Medical Students: Volume 1

94 ▶ D Carotid bodies primarily respond to hypoxia

A chemoreceptor is a receptor that responds to a change in the chemical composition of the blood. Chemoreceptors are the most important receptors involved in the minute-to-minute control of ventilation. There are both central and peripheral chemoreceptors.

Central chemoreceptors lie within the medulla of the brain stem. They primarily respond to hypercapnia by increasing the ventilatory rate and depth of ventilation.

Peripheral chemoreceptors lie in the carotid bodies (at the origin of the internal carotid artery) and the aortic arch. Carotid bodies must not be confused with the nearby carotid sinus baroreceptors, which are made up of stretch receptors in the wall of internal carotid arteries. Carotid bodies primarily respond to hypoxia by increasing the ventilatory rate and depth of ventilation.

Of the hypercapnic response driving ventilation, 80% arises from the central chemoreceptors and 20% from the peripheral chemoreceptors. The response of the central chemoreceptors to arterial $P(co_2)$ is therefore more important than that of the peripheral chemoreceptors. The hypoxic response driving ventilation comes almost entirely from the peripheral chemoreceptors.

Each carotid body is only a few millimetres in size and has the distinction of having the highest blood flow per tissue weight of any organ in the body (20 mL/g per min). This high flow is consistent with the prompt physiological reflex functions of the carotid body. Carotid bodies sample the partial pressure of oxygen in the blood, not its oxygen content. Anaemia, when the oxygen content is low but the $P(o_2)$ is normal, does not stimulate them.

95   C   The Haldane effect describes changes in the affinity of the blood for CO_2 with variations in the $Pa(o_2)$

Carbon dioxide is transported in the blood in three ways:

1. Bicarbonate accounts for about 80–90% of the total CO_2 in the blood.

2. Transported as carbamino compounds (5–10%).

3. Physically dissolved in solution (only 5%).

CO_2 is carried on the haemoglobin molecule as carbamino-haemoglobin; carboxyhaemoglobin is the combination of haemoglobin with carbon monoxide.

Venous blood contains a higher $P(co_2)$ than arterial blood and is therefore more acidic (through the formation of carbonic acid), with a lower pH.

CO_2 is approximately 20 times more soluble in plasma than O_2. This means that CO_2 diffuses about 20 times more rapidly than O_2. This rapid diffusion of CO_2 through aqueous solutions means that the elimination of CO_2 is much less of a problem than O_2 delivery, and therefore O_2 is likely to be the factor affected first in disorders of respiration.

Binding of O_2 with haemoglobin tends to displace CO_2 from the blood; this is known as the Haldane effect. In the capillaries, the Haldane effect causes increased pick-up of CO_2 because of the removal of O_2 from haemoglobin, whereas in the lungs it causes increased release of CO_2 because of the pick-up of O_2 by haemoglobin.

E Has a shape that is explained by the physicochemical properties of haemoglobin

The haemoglobin–oxygen dissociation curve is sigmoidal in shape. The sigmoid response reflects the underlying biochemical properties of haemoglobin and results from cooperativity, ie the protein cannot be considered in terms of four independently oxygen-binding subunits.

As haemoglobin binds successive oxygens, the oxygen affinity of the subunits increases. Hyperbolic curves are exhibited by monomeric molecules, such as myoglobin. The significance of the sigmoidal curve is that haemoglobin becomes highly saturated at high oxygen partial pressures (and is therefore highly efficient at collecting oxygen), and releases a significant amount of O_2 at pressures that are fairly low, but not extremely so (with the result that haemoglobin is highly effective at supplying O_2 where it is needed).

The effect of things that shift the curve to the right (raised CO_2, lowered pH, increased temperature, increase in 2,3-diphosphoglycerate or 2,3-DPG) is to increase O_2 availability in the tissues. The effect of CO_2/H^+ on O_2 carriage is known as the Bohr shift or effect. This is exactly what is needed in metabolising tissues; release of acids or CO_2 thus liberates O_2 to fulfil the metabolic needs of the tissue. Do not confuse this with the effect of changes in O_2 on CO_2 carriage, which is called the Haldane effect.

A shift of the oxygen dissociation curve to the left is characteristic of fetal haemoglobin. When compared with adult haemoglobin, it is composed of two α and two γ chains, instead of the usual two α and two β chains of adult haemoglobin. This arrangement assists in the transfer of oxygen across the placenta from the maternal to the fetal circulation. The corollary of this is that fetal tissue oxygen levels have to be low to permit the release of oxygen from the haemoglobin.

ANSWERS

Respiratory physiology – Answers

At high altitude, a decreased atmospheric pressure results in decreased ambient oxygen concentrations and therefore a decrease in arterial $P(o_2)$. In the short term, an increase in pulmonary ventilation occurs as a result of stimulation of peripheral chemoreceptors by lack of oxygen.

Hyperventilation causes a respiratory alkalosis (rise in arterial pH) by blowing off CO_2. This inhibits the central chemoreceptors and thereby opposes the effect of low $P(o_2)$ to stimulate the peripheral chemoreceptors (braking effect). Hypoxia leads to pulmonary vasoconstriction and pulmonary hypertension.

Acclimatisation (ie adaptive responses to sustained and gradually increasing hypoxia) occurs in the longer term through a variety of different mechanisms:

- Removal of the braking effect by changes in the composition of the cerebrospinal fluid (CSF) (a reduction in the bicarbonate concentration of the CSF) and increasing the renal excretion of bicarbonate. The result is increased pulmonary ventilation.

- Erythropoiesis through the effect of hypoxia stimulating erythropoietin secretion from the kidney. This increases the oxygen-carrying capacity of the blood, but in so doing raises blood haematocrit and blood viscosity, the effects of which can be deleterious.

- Increased cardiac output.

- Increased capillarity (increased number of capillaries in tissues).

- An increase in the concentration of 2,3-DPG – this causes a rightward shift of the O_2 dissociation curve that results in better unloading of O_2.

- Cellular acclimatisation – changes occur in the mitochondria and oxidative enzymes inside the cells.

If a person ascends to a high altitude too quickly (without giving enough time for these acclimatisation mechanisms to develop), or remains at high altitude for too long, high-altitude or mountain sickness may result. There is only one treatment for high-altitude sickness and that is immediate descent from the mountain.

98   B   Under resting conditions, equilibrium between alveolar $P(O_2)$ and red blood cells $P(CO_2)$ occurs one-third of the way along the pulmonary capillary

Gas exchange within the lung takes place at the level of the alveoli. It obeys Fick's law, which states that the rate of transfer of a gas through a sheet of tissue is directly proportional to the tissue surface area and the difference in partial pressures between the two sides, and is inversely proportional to the tissue thickness.

The area of the blood–gas barrier in the lung is enormous (50–100 m^2 – about the size of a tennis court) and its thickness is only $0.3\,\mu$m in some places, so the dimensions of the barrier are ideal for diffusion.

Any disruption to the factors that affect the rate of gas transfer through the respiratory membrane may result in disease states, eg the thickness of the respiratory membrane increases significantly in interstitial fibrosis, pulmonary oedema and pneumonia, interfering with the normal respiratory exchange of gases. Likewise, the surface area may be greatly decreased in emphysema, to name one example.

The capillaries form a dense network in the walls of the alveoli. The diameter of a capillary is just large enough for a red blood cell; this further increases the efficacy of gaseous exchange by reducing the distance required for diffusion to take place. At rest, each red blood cell spends, on average, about three-quarters of a second in the capillary network and during this time probably traverses two or three alveoli. Under typical resting conditions, the capillary $P(o_2)$ virtually reaches that of the alveolar gas (ie equilibration occurs) when the red cell is about one-third of the way along the capillary. This acts as a safety factor so that during exercise, when the time spent in the capillary by the red cell decreases, it does not compromise oxygenation.

Carbon monoxide (rather than chlorine gas) is the gas of choice for measuring the transfer factor (ie the effectiveness of the diffusing surface). Carbon monoxide is used in the test because its great avidity for haemoglobin means that its concentration in the blood can be assumed to be zero and does not need to be measured.

Compliance is expressed as volume change per unit change in pressure. Elastance is the reciprocal of compliance. Compliance is extremely small in infants compared with adults. The pressure–volume curve of the lung is non-linear with the lungs becoming stiffer at high volumes.

The curves that the lung follows in inflation and deflation are different. This behaviour is known as hysteresis. The lung volume at any given pressure during deflation is larger than that during inflation. This behaviour depends on structural proteins (collagen, elastin), surface tension and the surfactant's properties.

A sigh or yawn is a reflexly generated single deep breath that occurs after a period of quiet breathing. The purpose of the lung inflation, which stretches and unfolds the alveolar surface area, is to spread out the surfactant molecules, returning the alveolar surface tension to its normal value.

Various disease states are associated with either a decrease or an increase in lung compliance. Fibrosis, atelectasis and pulmonary oedema all result in a decrease in lung compliance (stiffer lungs). An increased lung compliance occurs in emphysema where an alteration in elastic tissue is probably responsible (secondary to the long-term effects of smoking). The lung effectively behaves like a 'soggy bag' so that a given pressure change results in a large change in volume (ie the lungs are more compliant). However, during expiration the airways are less readily supported and collapse at higher lung volumes, resulting in gas trapping and hyperinflation. Reduced gas transfer results from a loss of interstitial tissue causing loss of available active alveolar area.

100   C   Each haemoglobin molecule combines with eight oxygen atoms

Formation of haemoglobin:

1. Four pyrrole rings $\rightarrow$ protoporphyrin IX

2. Protoporphyrin IX + Fe^{2+} $\rightarrow$ haem

3. Haem + polypeptide (globin) $\rightarrow$ haemoglobin chain (α or β)

4. Two α chains + two β chains $\rightarrow$ haemoglobin A (normal adult Hb).

In normal adult haemoglobin, iron exists in the reduced, or ferrous (Fe^{2+}), state rather than the ferric (Fe^{3+}) state. Oxygen combines with the ferrous iron present within the haem molecules and not with the globin chains. The globin molecules that surround the haem molecule serve two key functions: they form a microenvironment in which the Fe^{2+} is protected from oxidation and also contribute to the unique oxygen-binding properties of haemoglobin (allosterism and cooperativity). When iron exists in the ferric, instead of the normal ferrous, state, the haemoglobin is known as methaemoglobin. This is abnormal and has a reduced oxygen-carrying capacity, resulting in cyanosis.

Haemoglobin consisting of two α and two γ chains is fetal haemoglobin. Normal adult haemoglobin contains two α and two β chains. As each haemoglobin chain has a haem prosthetic group, there are four iron atoms in each haemoglobin molecule. Each of these can bind with one molecule of oxygen, making a total of four molecules of oxygen (or eight oxygen atoms) that can be transported by each haemoglobin molecule.

Why do we have red blood cells?

- Primarily for the transport of haemoglobin and oxygen. If haemoglobin molecules were free in the plasma (and not wrapped up inside red cells) they would get filtered through the capillary membrane into the tissue spaces, or through the glomerular membrane, and would escape into the urine. For haemoglobin to remain in the bloodstream, it must exist inside red blood cells.

- There are enzyme systems in the red cell that help to prevent haemoglobin breakdown, eg methaemoglobin reductase converts ferric methaemoglobin (Fe^{3+}) back to ferrous (Fe^{2+}) haemoglobin.

- Carbonic anhydrase is restricted to the red cells and is crucial in CO_2 transport.

- The chemical environment in the cell, especially the presence of DPG, displaces the dissociation curve to the right so that oxygen unloads readily in active tissues.

- If haemoglobin were free in plasma, the viscosity of blood would rise to intolerable levels and colloid osmotic pressure would increase considerably. The viscosity effect is especially important in capillaries where the presence of red cells in blood gives it an anomalously low viscosity (Fahraeus–Lindqvist effect).

Renal physiology
Answers

101 **D** Acts via a secondary messenger

Erythropoietin is a glycoprotein hormone, produced mainly by the juxtaglomerular apparatus of the kidney in adults. In the fetus, it is almost solely produced by the liver.

Once released, erythropoietin acts on specific receptors, which leads to activation of tyrosine kinase; this, in turn, promotes transcription towards the manufacture of more red cells from bone marrow.

The major factor causing erythropoietin release is local hypoxia in the kidney, which may derive from anaemia or systemic hypoxia. Erythropoietin secretion is a prominent feature of acclimatisation to high altitude. A deficiency of erythropoietin partly explains the anaemia seen in individuals with chronic renal failure. Recombinant erythropoietin is now available, revolutionising treatment.

B Production is decreased by angiotensin-converting enzyme inhibitors

Aldosterone is a steroid hormone secreted by the zona glomerulosa layer of the adrenal cortex. Secretion continues after the removal of the kidneys and their juxtaglomerular cells because factors other than the renin–angiotensin system result in the secretion of aldosterone (eg hyperkalaemia).

Angiotensin-converting enzyme (ACE) inhibitors tend to reduce the level of angiotensin II, which normally stimulates the adrenal cortex to produce aldosterone. The reduction of angiotensin II and aldosterone in part explains the antihypertensive effect of ACE inhibitors.

Aldosterone increases the excretion of both potassium and hydrogen ions from the distal convoluted tubule and collecting ducts. This results in a potassium diuresis and acidic urine of a low pH.

C Activation results in the stimulation of aldosterone release

Renin   ACE (in lungs)

↓   ↓

Angiotensinogen → Angiotensin I → Angiotensin II

Angiotensinogen is synthesised by the liver; renin catalyses the production of angiotensin I (a decapeptide) from angiotensinogen. Angiotensin I is further cleaved to an octapeptide, angiotensin II, by ACE, which is found mainly in the capillaries of the lungs. Collectively, this is known as the renin–angiotensin system.

The effects of activation of the renin–angiotensin system are severalfold:

- Stimulation of aldosterone release from the adrenal cortex; this increases sodium and water retention, helping to maintain the arterial pressure.

- Enhanced NaCl and water reabsorption from the proximal convoluted tubule.

- Widespread vasoconstriction caused by angiotensin; this increases the systemic vascular resistance and therefore the arterial pressure. The resulting vasoconstriction also reduces the GFR at a time when water has to be conserved.

- Stimulation of ADH secretion from the posterior pituitary: leads to an increased solute-free water reabsorption.

- Stimulation of thirst (dipsogenic effect).

104 **D A fall in pressure in the afferent arteriole promotes renin secretion**

The juxtaglomerular apparatus is a specialisation of the glomerular afferent arteriole and the distal convoluted tubule of the corresponding nephron; it is involved in the regulation of extracellular volume and blood pressure via the renin–angiotensin system.

The juxtaglomerular apparatus is composed of three components:

1. Macula densa: specialised epithelial cells lining the distal convoluted tubule.

2. Juxtaglomerular cells (also known as granular cells) of the afferent arterioles: modified smooth muscle cells that are renin secreting.

3. Extraglomerular mesangial cells (also known as Lacis cells or Goormaghtigh cells): their function remains obscure. They contain contractile proteins that are instrumental in the fine-tuning of glomerular filtration. They have phagocytic properties and may act as antigen-presenting cells; they may also be the site of secretion of the hormone erythropoietin.

The renin–angiotensin system is triggered to release renin in three circumstances:

1. Fall in the renal perfusion pressure detected by baroreceptors in the afferent arterioles.

2. Activation of the sympathetic nervous system: occurs when there is a fall in arterial blood pressure.

3. Reduced sodium delivery to the macula densa (as detected by osmoreceptors): occurs when there is also a fall in renal perfusion pressure. An unknown paracrine factor is believed

to act between the macula densa and juxtaglomerular cells to stimulate renin release (a prostaglandin or nitric oxide has been postulated).

The renin–angiotensin system is strongly implicated in the pathogenesis of hypertension secondary to renal artery stenosis. The juxtaglomerular apparatus of the affected kidney responds to decreased perfusion pressure by increasing renin secretion (Goldblatt's hypertension).

105 A Increases in response to a $\geq$ 10% loss of circulatory volume

Antidiuretic hormone (ADH) synthesis occurs in the cell bodies of the magnocellular neurons in the supraoptic (5/6) and paraventricular nuclei (1/6) of the hypothalamus. From there, ADH is transported down the axons of these neurons to their endings in the posterior pituitary (neurohypophysis or pars nervosa), where they are stored as secretory granules before release. Release is controlled directly by nerve impulses passing down the axons from the hypothalamus; this process is known as neurosecretion.

Increased secretion of ADH occurs in response to two main stimuli: an increase in plasma osmolality and a decrease in the effective circulating volume. Significant changes in secretion occur when osmolality is changed as little as 1%. Such a change is detected by osmoreceptors that lie outside the blood–brain barrier and appear to be located in the circumventricular organs, particularly the organum vasculosum of the lamina terminalis. In this way, the osmoreceptors rapidly respond to changes in plasma osmolality and in normal individuals plasma osmolality is maintained very close to 285 mOsmol/L. ADH secretion is considerably more sensitive to small changes in osmolality than to similar changes in blood volume. Plasma ADH levels do not increase appreciably until blood volume is reduced by about 10%, when ADH plays a significant role in the response to haemorrhage.

ADH has two main actions: it increases free water absorption from the collecting ducts of the kidney (thereby conserving water) and is a potent vasoconstrictor. The mechanism by which ADH exerts its antidiuretic effect is through the action on V2 receptors and insertion of protein water channels (aquaporins) in the luminal membranes of collecting duct cells. Aquaporins are stored in endosomes inside cells and ADH causes their translocation to the cell membrane via a cAMP pathway. In this way, the urine becomes concentrated and its volume decreases in response to an increase in plasma osmolality and a rise in ADH; this osmoregulatory action of ADH is a good example of a homoeostatic mechanism. Vasoconstriction is mediated via V1 receptors, as well as the phosphoinositol pathway. The latter effect has an important role in maintaining arterial blood pressure in haemorrhagic shock.

Hypersecretion of ADH occurs in the syndrome of inappropriate ADH release (SIADH). Diabetes insipidus is the syndrome that results when there is ADH deficiency (cranial form), or the kidney fails to respond to the hormone (nephrogenic form). It should not to be confused with diabetes mellitus; the term 'diabetes' is derived from the Greek meaning siphon, and simply reflects the excessive passing of urine in both conditions.

D The kidney is able to generate new bicarbonate from glutamine

The precision with which H^+ concentration is regulated emphasises its importance to the various cell functions. The normal pH of the blood is held remarkably constant within the limits 7.35–7.45. It is essential that the pH be kept within these stringent limits in order to prevent the denaturation of body proteins and enzymes. This is yet another example of homoeostasis, whereby the constancy of the 'internal milieu' is essential to life.

There are three primary systems that regulate the pH in the body:

1. The chemical buffer systems of the body fluids.
2. The respiratory system (which regulates the removal of CO_2 and therefore carbonic acid from the blood).
3. The kidneys.

The bone and liver also have a small role to play in the regulation of pH. When there is a change in pH, the buffer systems work fastest (within a fraction of a second) to minimise the change in pH. Of these, the bicarbonate buffer system is the most important extracellular buffer. The second line of defence is the respiratory system, which acts within a few minutes. These first two lines of defence keep the pH constant until the more slowly responding third line of defence, the kidneys, can eliminate the excess acid or base from the body. Although the kidneys are relatively slow to respond compared with the other defences (taking hours to days), they are the most powerful of the acid–base regulatory systems.

The renal tubule actively secretes H^+ and reabsorbs HCO_3^-. Acute renal failure therefore results in an inability to excrete acid and metabolic acidosis. There are three main methods by which the kidney absorbs HCO_3^-:

1. Replacement of filtered HCO_3^- with HCO_3^- that is generated in tubular cells.

2. The generation of new HCO_3^- by the phosphate buffer system, which carries excess H^+ into the urine.

3. The generation of new HCO_3^- from glutamine molecules that are absorbed by the tubular cell (the ammonia buffer system).

 107 ▶ **D** The low blood flow in the vasa recta assists in the formation of a concentrated urine

In a normal adult human the combined blood flow through both kidneys is about 1200 mL/min, or about 20% of the cardiac output. Considering that the kidneys constitute only about 0.4% of total body weight, they receive an extremely high blood flow compared with other tissues.

The high flow to the kidney greatly exceeds the metabolic demands (the kidneys account for only 6% of total oxygen consumption). The purpose of this additional flow is to supply enough plasma for the high rates of glomerular filtration that are necessary for precise regulation of body fluid volumes and solute concentrations. The organic acid, *p*-aminohippuric acid, has traditionally been used to measure renal blood flow.

The kidneys have effective mechanisms for maintaining the constancy of renal blood flow and GFR over an arterial pressure range between 70 and 170 mmHg – a process called autoregulation. This helps to maintain a normal excretion of metabolic waste products, such as urea and creatinine, which depend on GFR for their excretion. Autoregulation is an intrinsic property of the kidney; therefore transplanted kidneys will autoregulate. There are two main theories to explain how renal autoregulation of blood flow occurs: tubuloglomerular feedback and the myogenic mechanism.

Angiotensin II preferentially constricts the efferent more than the afferent arteriole. This has the effect of raising glomerular filtration pressure, while reducing renal blood flow. Under circumstances of decreased arterial blood pressure (when angiotensin II is released), this helps to prevent decreases in GFR (tubuloglomerular feedback method of autoregulation); at the same time, by reducing renal blood flow, it causes increased reabsorption of sodium and water. In cases of renal artery stenosis, maintenance of the glomerular filtration pressure is dependent on the angiotensin II-dependent vasoconstriction of the efferent arteriole. Administration of ACE inhibitors abolishes the vasoconstriction of the efferent arteriole, resulting in an abrupt fall in the GFR. This explains why ACE inhibitors are contraindicated in renal artery stenosis.

Flow to the renal medulla is supplied by long capillary loops called the vasa recta. These descend into the medulla in parallel with the loops of Henle. The blood flow in them is very low compared with flow in the renal cortex. This helps to maintain the hyperosmotic medullary interstitial gradient, thereby assisting in the formation of concentrated urine.

108 ▶ D The glomerular filtration barrier comprises three layers

In the normal adult human the GFR (or normal renal clearance) averages 125 mL/min, or 180 L/day. The entire plasma volume (about 3 L) can therefore be filtered and processed by the kidney approximately 60 times every day. The rate of urine production in humans is dominated by tubular function, not GFR, which remains relatively constant through autoregulation.

After the age of 35 years, the GFR falls at about 1 mL/min per year. By the age of 80, the GFR has fallen to about 50% of its youthful level, and it can decrease by as much as 50% before plasma creatinine rises beyond the normal range. Consequently, a normal creatinine does not necessarily imply normal renal function, although a raised creatinine usually indicates impaired renal function.

A substance used to measure the GFR must be freely filtered at the glomerulus, not secreted by the tubules, not reabsorbed, not metabolised or synthesised in the body, non-toxic and soluble in plasma, and something that does not alter the renal function/ GFR. Such a substance is the polyfructose molecule, inulin. However, it is too cumbersome to use in routine clinical practice. Instead, GFR is more commonly quantified by measuring the 24-hour urinary creatinine excretion. p-Aminohippuric acid is used to measure renal blood flow and not GFR.

The glomerular filtration barrier comprises three layers:

1. The capillary endothelium

2. Basement membrane

3. Layer of epithelial cells (podocytes).

From the anatomy of the glomerulus, it is clear that the 'actual filter' (and the primary restriction point for proteins) is the basement membrane layer.

ANSWERS

MCQs in Applied Basic Sciences for Medical Students: Volume 1

230

E   The maximum concentrating ability of the human kidney is 1200 mOsmol/L

The filtered load of glucose normally undergoes complete reabsorption in the proximal convoluted tubule (remember the most important substances for survival are generally absorbed first). Therefore, no glucose is usually found in the urine. However, when the filtered load exceeds the capacity of the tubules to reabsorb glucose (as in uncontrolled diabetes mellitus), urinary excretion of glucose occurs (glycosuria).

Of sodium reabsorption 70% takes place in the proximal convoluted tubule, 20% in the ascending limb of the loop of Henle and only 10% in the distal convoluted tubule and collecting ducts. It is only the last that is aldosterone dependent.

The maximum concentration of urine that can be excreted by the human kidney is 1200 mOsmol/L – four times the osmolality of plasma. This is primarily a function of the length of the loop of Henle, the hyperosmotic medullary interstitial gradient and the concentration of ADH. A countercurrent multiplication system sets up an osmotic gradient in the renal medulla, which allows an efficient way for urine to be concentrated over a relatively short distance along the nephron with minimal energy expenditure. The descending limb of the loop of Henle is permeable to water (but only slightly permeable to salt and urea). Therefore, water is progressively absorbed down the limb, becoming more and more concentrated (up to 1200 mOsmol/L). The ascending limb is impermeable to water, but permeable to sodium chloride. The tubular fluid is therefore hypotonic by the time it reaches the distal convoluted tubule and collecting ducts. In the presence of a high concentration of ADH, by the time the urine is excreted it has a high osmolality (of up to 1200 mOsmol/L).

ANSWERS

Renal physiology – Answers

The limited ability of the human kidney to concentrate urine to a maximal concentration of 1200 mOsmol/L helps to explain why severe dehydration occurs on drinking seawater. The osmolality of seawater averages 2400 mOsmol/L, so drinking 1 litre of seawater would give a total solute concentration of 2400 mOsmol. If the maximal urine-concentrating ability of the human kidney were 1200 mOsmol/L, 2 litres would be required to rid the body of these solutes. This would result in a net loss of 1 L for every litre of seawater drunk, explaining the rapid dehydration that occurs in shipwreck victims who drink seawater. In short, if lost at sea, you are better off drinking nothing than drinking seawater.

Gastrointestinal physiology Answers

110   **D**   It is richer in potassium than any other gastrointestinal secretion

The salivary glands can be divided into the major (parotid, submandibular and sublingual) glands and minor glands:

- Parotid secretion is mainly serous.
- Submandibular secretion is mainly mixed (mucinous and serous).
- Sublingual secretion is mainly mucinous.

In humans about 1–1.5 L of saliva are secreted each day. In the unstimulated state, most of the saliva originates from the submandibular gland but when active most of it arises from the parotid gland. Secretion is an active process. The two-stage hypothesis of salivation states that a primary secretion is first formed by secretory end-pieces (which resembles an ultrafiltrate of plasma), which is then modified as it flows along the duct system. Na^+ and Cl^- are absorbed and K^+ and HCO_3^- are secreted as saliva flows along the ductal system. In addition, the ducts have a low water permeability. The final saliva is hypotonic with respect to plasma and contains a higher K^+ concentration than any other gastrointestinal secretion of the body.

Saliva contains principally water, mucus, enzymes (mainly salivary amylase, lingual lipase and the antibacterial enzyme lysozyme), antibodies and inorganic ions. It does not contain trypsin, which is secreted by the exocrine pancreas.

Sialolithiasis (stone formation) may occur in any major salivary gland but is most common in the submandibular gland. There are two reasons for this phenomenon. The submandibular saliva is rich in mucus and is, thus, more viscous than parotid saliva. In addition the submandibular duct ascends against gravity when the body is upright, bends at the posterior edge of the mouth, and takes a long and tortuous course. This means that there is a particular tendency in this gland to secretory congestion and calculus formation.

Goblet cells are mucus-secreting cells widely distributed in epithelial surfaces, but especially dense in the gastrointestinal and respiratory tracts.

Kupffer cells have phagocytic properties and are found in the liver. They participate in the removal of ageing erythrocytes and other particulate debris.

The gastric mucosa contains many cell subtypes including acid-secreting cells (also known as parietal or oxyntic cells), pepsin-secreting cells (also known as peptic, chief or zymogenic cells) and G-cells (gastrin-secreting cells). Peptic cells synthesise and secrete the proteolytic enzyme pepsin. Parietal cells actively secrete hydrochloric acid into the gastric lumen, accounting for the acidic environment encountered in the stomach. However, parietal cells are also involved in the secretion of the glycoprotein, intrinsic factor.

Intrinsic factor plays a pivotal role in the absorption of vitamin B_{12} from the terminal ileum. Autoimmune attack against parietal cells leads to a lack of intrinsic factor and hydrochloric acid, in turn leading to vitamin B_{12} deficiency and achlorhydria. This is known as pernicious anaemia.

ANSWERS

Gastrointestinal physiology – Answers

112 ▶ B Is potentiated by histamine

There are three classic phases of gastric acid secretion:

1. Cephalic (preparatory) phase (significant): results in the production of gastric acid before food actually enters the stomach. It is triggered by the sight, smell, thought and taste of food acting via the vagus nerve.

2. Gastric phase (most significant): initiated by the presence of food in the stomach, particularly protein-rich food.

3. Intestinal phase (least significant): the presence of amino acids and food in the duodenum stimulate acid production.

Gastric acid is stimulated by three factors:

1. Acetylcholine: from parasympathetic neurons of the vagus nerve that innervate parietal cells directly.

2. Gastrin: produced by pyloric G-cells.

3. Histamine: produced by mast cells. This stimulates the parietal cells directly and also potentiates parietal cell stimulation by gastrin and neuronal stimulation. H_2-receptor blockers such as ranitidine are therefore an effective way of reducing acid secretion.

Gastric acid is inhibited by three factors:

1. Somatostatin

2. Secretin

3. Cholecystokinin.

Gastrin is secreted by gastrin-secreting cells (G-cells) found in two locations: the pyloric region of the stomach and the upper half of the small intestine.

Gastrin is released by:

- vagal stimulation
- distension of the pyloric antrum
- proteins (especially partially digested proteins) in the food.

Gastrin is inhibited by:

- a low pH in the lumen of the pyloric antrum (negative feedback loop)
- somatostatin.

Gastrin has three main actions:

1. Stimulates gastric acid secretion
2. Stimulates gastric motility
3. Stimulates exocrine pancreatic secretions.

Overproduction of gastrin leads to excessive gastric acid secretion and the formation of multiple peptic ulcers. This is known as the Zollinger–Ellison syndrome and is often the result of a gastrin-secreting tumour (gastrinoma).

114 ▶ D Has its main stimulation for secretion during the intestinal phase

The pancreas is a mixed endocrine (ductless) and exocrine gland that forms embyologically from the fusion of separate dorsal and ventral pancreatic buds (endodermal outgrowths from the primitive foregut). The embryology helps to explain how aberrations of development lead to the formation of an annular pancreas, or pancreas divisum, either of which may lead to problems in later life.

The exocrine component of the pancreas consists of closely packed secretory acini, which drain into a highly branched duct system. Approximately 1500 mL of pancreatic juice is secreted each day into the duodenum via the pancreatic duct. The alkaline pH of the pancreatic secretion (about 8.0) is a result of a high content of HCO_3^- and serves to neutralise the acidic chyme as it enters the duodenum from the stomach.

As for the secretion of gastric acid, it is possible to distinguish cephalic, gastric and intestinal phases in the pattern of secretion. The weak cephalic phase contributes only 15% of the total response, an enzyme-rich secretion caused by vagal efferents. The weak gastric phase also contributes only 15% of the total response and is again enzyme rich, caused by vasovagal reflexes originating in the stomach and gastrin secretion. The main stimulation (70% of the total response) is the intestinal phase caused by food entering the duodenum from the stomach. Secretin, a hormone released by endocrine cells scattered in the duodenal mucosa, promotes the secretion of copious watery fluid rich in HCO_3^-. The major stimulus for the release of secretin is acid. Cholecystokinin, also derived from duodenal endocrine cells, stimulates the secretion of enzyme-rich pancreatic fluid. Secretin and cholecystokinin act synergistically.

115   A   Trypsin is a powerful activator of other pancreatic proteolytic enzymes

The pancreatic enzymes degrade proteins, carbohydrates, lipids and nucleic acids. The pancreatic proteolytic enzymes, trypsin and chymotrypsin, are secreted as inactive proenzymes that require activation in the small intestine.

Enterokinase (enteropeptidase), an enzyme secreted by the duodenal mucosa, activates trypsinogen to form trypsin; trypsin then activates chymotrypsinogen to form chymotrypsin and other proenzymes into active enzymes. Trypsin can also activate trypsinogen, so, once some trypsin is formed, there is an autocatalytic chain reaction. By releasing the enzymes as inactive zymogens that become activated far from their site of origin, this mechanism prevents autodigestion of the pancreas.

The powerful nature of these proteolytic enzymes, however, necessitates another mechanism to prevent digestion of the pancreas. The same cells that secrete the proteolytic enzymes also secrete another substance called trypsin inhibitor (not a trypsin activator, which would be disastrous!). Trypsin inhibitor surrounds the enzyme granules and prevents activation of trypsin both inside the secretory cells and in the acini and ducts of the pancreas. It therefore acts as an additional safeguard should some of the trypsinogen be activated to trypsin. After exocytosis this inhibitor is diluted out and becomes ineffective. As trypsin activates the other pancreatic proteolytic enzymes too, trypsin inhibitor therefore prevents the subsequent activation of the others as well.

When the pancreas becomes severely damaged or when the duct becomes blocked, large quantities of pancreatic secretion become pooled in the damaged areas of the pancreas. Under these circumstances, the effect of trypsin inhibitor is overwhelmed, in which case the pancreatic secretions rapidly

ANSWERS

Gastrointestinal physiology – Answers

become activated and literally digest the entire pancreas, giving rise to a condition known as acute pancreatitis. This can be lethal; even if not fatal, it may lead to a lifetime of pancreatic insufficiency.

116 ▸ C   Islets of Langerhans make up only 2% of volume of the gland

The endocrine tissue of the pancreas forms the islets of Langerhans. They make up about 2% of the volume of the pancreas, whereas the exocrine portion makes up 80% and ducts and blood vessels make up the rest. Pancreatic endocrine tissue, like all endocrine tissue, is ductless.

There are several different types of islet cell, each producing a different hormone:

- α-islet cells secrete glucagon
- β-islet cells secrete insulin
- δ-islet cells secrete somatostatin
- F-islet cells secrete pancreatic polypeptide.

Each of these hormones passes directly into the bloodstream.

Glucagon has a reciprocal action to that of insulin. It is glycogenolytic, gluconeogenic, lipolytic and ketogenic.

The liver secretes about 500 mL of alkaline bile daily. It is composed of 97% water, 0.7% bile salts (sodium and potassium salts of bile acids), 0.2% bile pigments (bilirubin and biliverdin) and 2% other substances (bicarbonate, fatty acids, cholesterol, lecithin).

Bile salts are derived from cholesterol – do not confuse them with bile pigments, which are the breakdown products of the haem component of haemoglobin. In addition it is the accumulation of bile pigments (bilirubin) that leads to jaundice.

Bile salts are responsible for the emulsification of fat in the chyme, by the formation of micelles. This aids in their absorption. Bile contains no digestive enzymes.

Of the bile salts, 90–95% are absorbed from the small intestine and then excreted again from the liver; most are absorbed from the terminal ileum. This is known as the enterohepatic circulation. The entire pool recycles twice per meal and about six to eight times per day. Disruption of the enterohepatic circulation, either by terminal ileal resection or through a diseased terminal ileum (eg Crohn's disease), results in decreased fat absorption and cholesterol gallstone formation. The latter is believed to result because bile salts normally make cholesterol more water soluble through the formation of cholesterol micelles.

Between meals the sphincter of Oddi, which guards the opening of the bile duct into the duodenum, is constricted and bile passes into the gallbladder. The gallbladder serves three main functions. It concentrates bile (5- to 20-fold) by the active reabsorption of salt and water through the gallbladder epithelium. It also stores bile and secretes mucus into the bile. The periodic discharge of bile from the gallbladder aids digestion but is not essential for it.

ANSWERS

Gastrointestinal physiology – Answers

Every day 7–10 L of water enter the alimentary canal. Most of this is absorbed by the end of the small intestine, so that only 500–600 mL enter the colon. Further reabsorption occurs in the colon so that only about 100 mL are lost from the body in the faeces.

Glucose absorption is dependent on sodium absorption, via a sodium (secondary active) co-transport mechanism. Conversely, the presence of glucose in the intestinal lumen facilitates the absorption of sodium. Water follows by osmosis. This is the physiological basis for the treatment of sodium and water loss in diarrhoea by oral administration of solutions containing sodium chloride and glucose (oral rehydration therapy). Most of the ingested sodium is reabsorbed (normally < 0.5% of intestinal sodium is lost in the faeces) because of its rapid absorption through the intestinal mucosa. If absorption is greater than the body requirements, the excess is excreted by the kidneys.

A good way to think about the order of absorption of substances throughout the gastrointestinal tract is to remember that the most important substances for survival are generally absorbed first, followed by the less important ones. Thus, glucose absorption takes place mainly in the upper small intestine (duodenum and jejunum), but vitamin B_{12} is absorbed further down, in the terminal ileum (as bodily stores of vitamin B_{12} can last up to 2 years in its complete absence).

Iron is absorbed more readily in the ferrous state (Fe^{2+}), but most of the dietary iron is in the ferric (Fe^{3+}) form. Gastric acidity releases iron from the food and favours the ferrous form, which is absorbed more easily. The importance of this function in humans is indicated by the fact that iron deficiency anaemia is a troublesome and relatively frequent complication of partial gastrectomy.

Starvation is a chronic state resulting from inadequate intake of energy. Four main metabolic processes occur during starvation: glycogenolysis, gluconeogenesis, lipolysis and ketogenesis. No significant hypoglycaemic episodes occur until the end stage of starvation is entered.

During the immediate phase of starvation (0–24 hours), reserves of glycogen from liver and skeletal muscle are used. Glucose produced from glycogen lasts only 24 hours. The blood glucose is maintained after glycogen is depleted by gluconeogenesis, for which the main substrates are amino acids, lactic acid and glycerol.

In general, fats spare nitrogen so that protein is preserved until relatively late in starvation. During prolonged starvation, ketone bodies (acetone, acetoacetate, β-hydroxybutyrate) derived from fats are used by the brain and other tissues (such as heart muscle). Although the brain is usually heavily dependent on glucose as its energy source, during starvation it adapts to using ketones.

When fat stores are finally used up, protein catabolism increases and death follows from proteolysis of vital muscles (cardiac muscle, diaphragm). The average time to death is about 60 days.

ANSWERS

Endocrine physiology and thermoregulation
Answers

120 ▶ **C Thyroid-stimulating hormone (TSH)**

The pituitary gland (hypophysis) is the conductor of the endocrine orchestra. It is divided into both an anterior part and a posterior part. The anterior pituitary (adenohypophysis or pars distalis) secretes six hormones, namely:

1. FSH (follicle-stimulating hormone): reproduction
2. LH (luteinising hormone): reproduction
3. ACTH (adrenocorticotrophic hormone): stress response
4. TSH (thyroid-stimulating hormone): basal metabolic rate
5. GH (growth hormone): growth
6. Prolactin: lactation.

The posterior pituitary (neurohypophysis or pars nervosa) secretes only two hormones:

1. ADH (anti diuretic hormone) (vasopressin): osmotic regulation
2. Oxytocin: milk ejection and labour.

Testosterone is produced from Leydig cells in the testis and from the adrenal glands. Corticotrophin-releasing hormone (CRH) is produced by the median eminence of the hypothalamus.

 121 D Identical twins show 90% concordance

In type 1 diabetes mellitus identical twins have a 50% concordance, whereas in type 2 there is 90% concordance. Type 1 diabetes is associated with HLA-DR-3/-4, whereas type 2 diabetes has no HLA association. Type 1 diabetes is a disorder of insulin deficiency and therefore presentation is with weight loss and ketone production, usually early in life in the teenage years. In type 2 diabetes, which commonly presents after the age of 40, there is an association with obesity and insulin resistance rather than insulin deficiency itself.

122 C A fasting glucose of 7.5 mmol/L on two occasions is consistent with a diagnosis

It is vital to be aware of the diagnostic criteria for diabetes. A fasting glucose of > 7 mmol/L, or a glucose of > 11.1 mmol/L, 2 hours after a 75 g glucose load is diagnostic. A random glucose of > 11.1 mmol/L is also consistent with a diagnosis. One abnormal laboratory value is diagnostic in symptomatic individuals; two abnormal values are needed in asymptomatic individuals.

Impaired glucose tolerance is defined as a glucose level of 7.8–11.1 mmol/L 2 hours after 75 g glucose and impaired fasting glucose is defined as a fasting glucose level of > 6 and < 7 mmol/L.

123

D It is an anabolic hormone

Insulin acts via cell membrane-spanning receptors that have intrinsic receptor tyrosine kinase activity. When insulin binds to the receptor, the tyrosine kinase is phosphorylated, resulting in a cascade of intracellular signalling mechanisms, which in turn results in glucose uptake into the cell. It is secreted by β cells of the pancreas.

Somatostatin is secreted by δ cells. Secretion is inhibited by somatostatin, which is always considered an inhibitory hormone. Insulin is considered an anabolic hormone, ie it takes up glucose into the cell and converts it into larger 'building blocks' such as proteins and fats. Release of insulin is stimulated not only by the ingestion of glucose but also by amino acids that it will convert into larger proteins.

124

B Prolactin is under dominant inhibitary regulation

Oxytocin and ADH are synthesised in the paraventricular and supraoptic nuclei of the hypothalamus. They are transported from the hypothalamus down into the posterior pituitary gland (or neurohypophysis) via magnocellular neurons and are stored in the posterior pituitary as vesicles before release into the bloodstream.

GH, ACTH, TSH, prolactin and leuteinising hormone (LH)/FSH are released from the anterior pituitary gland. Prolactin is under inhibitory control by dopamine, but can also be stimulated by thyroid hormone-releasing hormone (TRH)/TSH. Catecholamines, serotonin and T_4 are amine hormones, whereas cortisol, aldosterone, androgens, oestrogens, progesterone and vitamin D are steroid hormones. All other hormones are peptide hormones.

Insulin, GH and prolactin act via tyrosine kinase receptors. Epinephrine, ACTH, TSH, LH/FSH, glucagon and somatostatin act via G-protein receptors coupled to cAMP. The G-protein-coupled receptor activates adenylyl cyclase, which in turn generates cAMP in an amplification process. Gonadotrophin-releasing hormone (GnRH) and TRH act via G-protein receptors coupled to intracellular calcium as a second messenger. This is undertaken through activation of phospholipase C. It is the steroid hormones that bind to intracellular receptors.

125 ▶ E Has a peak hormonal concentration in the morning

Cortisol is a steroid hormone that is released in stress to cause an increase in blood glucose. It is a catabolic hormone and is stimulated by ACTH released from the anterior pituitary.

ACTH is stimulated by CRH released from the median eminence of the hypothalamus. It has a diurnal variation and peaks on waking up in the morning. Its lowest level is around midnight and this is why a 'midnight cortisol' is used to detect excess cortisol production in Cushing's syndrome.

126

D PTH acts directly on osteoblasts in bone

Four hormones are primarily concerned with the regulation of calcium metabolism:

1. PTH

2. Activated vitamin D (1,25-dihydroxycholecalciferol)

3. Calcitonin (secreted from the parafollicular cells [also known as the clear or C-cells] of the thyroid gland; relatively unimportant in humans).

4. Parathyroid hormone-related protein (PTHrP) – important in the hypercalcaemia of malignancy.

The main regulatory tissues are bone, the kidney and the intestine.

The 25-hydroxylation step of vitamin D activation occurs in the liver, whereas the 1-hydroxylation step occurs in the kidney. Activation of vitamin D requires both activation steps and PTH.

Effects of activated vitamin D:

- Intestine: 1,25-dihydroxycholecalciferol promotes the intestinal absorption of calcium and phosphate. Absence leads to rickets in children and osteomalacia in adults.

- Kidneys: increases tubular reabsorption of calcium and phosphate.

- Bone: mobilisation of calcium and phosphate.

PTH is secreted from the chief cells (also known as principal cells) of the parathyroid glands. The major regulator of PTH secretion is extracellular calcium. Circulating ionised calcium acts directly on the parathyroid glands in a negative feedback fashion to regulate the secretion of PTH. The pituitary gland does not play a role in the secretion of PTH.

ANSWERS

Endocrine physiology and thermoregulation – Answers

Effects of PTH:

- Bone: resorption with calcium and phosphate release into the bloodstream. PTH acts directly on osteoblasts and osteocytes that contain membrane receptors for PTH. Osteoclasts do not themselves have membrane receptors for PTH. Instead, it is believed that the activated osteoblasts and osteocytes send a secondary but 'unknown' paracrine signal to the osteoclasts, causing them to resorb bone.

- Kidney: PTH acts on the kidneys to increase calcium reabsorption and increase phosphate excretion (phosphaturic effect). There is one caveat to this: although PTH enhances renal calcium reabsorption, in hyperparathyroidism urinary calcium excretion is paradoxically increased because the reabsorbing mechanism is saturated. This increases the tendency to renal stone formation in hyperparathyroidism.

- Intestine: PTH increases the formation of activated vitamin D and this increases calcium absorption from the gut.

127

C **T$_4$ promotes the growth and development of the brain**

The thyroid gland primarily produces T$_4$ which is converted to T$_3$ (the more active form) in the periphery. T$_4$ is released when TSH, produced from the anterior pituitary, binds to cell surface receptors on the thyroid gland.

Thyroid hormone-releasing hormone (TRH) is a hypothalamic hormone that causes TSH secretion. TSH release is under inhibitory control by dopamine. T$_4$ increases basal metabolic rate. Metabolism of protein, carbohydrate and fat is increased. T$_4$, although not a steroid, does not act on cell surface receptors, but acts on intracellular receptors bound to promoters of genes. It directly affects gene transcription in this way. It plays an extremely important role in the myelination of axons during brain development. Neonatal deficiency leads to reduced axonal conduction velocities at the critical time in development when the brain is growing and maturing, resulting in developmental delay and mental handicap. This is known as cretinism or congenital hypothyroidism. Thyroid replacement therapy must be initiated soon after birth if mental handicap is to be prevented. Affected infants should be identified on neonatal biochemical screening (the Guthrie test).

Diabetic ketoacidosis results from insulin deficiency. Insulin is normally responsible for the uptake of glucose by cells in the body. Most of the pathological features can be attributed to one of the following effects of insulin lack:

- hyperglycaemia in the blood
- intracellular glucose deficiency.

A good way of thinking about diabetic ketoacidosis is, therefore, 'starvation in the midst of plenty'.

Insulin deficiency results in lipolysis, glycogenolysis, gluconeogenesis and ketogenesis, in an analogous way to starvation. The production of ketone bodies results in acetone breath and metabolic acidosis, with a fall in blood pH. The resulting acidosis stimulates the respiratory centre. This leads to a characteristic breathing pattern seen in diabetic ketoacidosis known as Kussmaul's breathing. Glucose spills over into the urine (glycosuria) when glucose levels exceed the capacity of the kidneys to reabsorb glucose. This produces an osmotic diuresis (with consequent polyuria and polydipsia).

The overall effect is a massive loss of fluid in the urine causing dehydration and circulatory collapse. Dehydration is worsened by the vomiting and hyperventilation that may also occur. Circulatory failure in itself worsens the metabolic acidosis (through lactic acidosis, acute renal failure, etc.) and leads to uraemia. A vicious cycle is set up leading to coma and death.

Insulin is normally responsible for driving potassium into cells, so insulin deficiency results in hyperkalaemia. This is worsened by any dehydration, metabolic acidosis or renal impairment from circulatory failure, which may also be present. Despite the hyperkalaemia, total body potassium content is actually low (secondary to vomiting, renal losses, etc).

The aims of treatment in diabetic ketoacidosis are threefold: insulin replacement, rehydration with intravenous fluids and potassium replacement. The last requires special attention; although potassium is initially high, when insulin is given potassium is rapidly driven into cells, resulting in hypokalaemia. Potassium therefore needs to be cautiously and judiciously replaced during the treatment of ketoacidosis.

129 ▶ E Congenital adrenal hyperplasia (adrenogenital syndrome) results in virilisation and salt wasting

Disorders of the adrenal gland may relate to the adrenal cortex or the medulla, or both. There is only one disorder worth mentioning that selectively affects the adrenal medulla – a phaeochromocytoma, which is a tumour of the adrenal medulla that results in the overproduction of catecholamines (such as epinephrine and norepinephrine). This leads to hypertension, headaches, palpitations and sweating (all known effects of epinephrine).

Conditions of the adrenal cortex may result from over- or underproduction of hormones. An overproduction of cortisol is known as Cushing's syndrome. There are several causes of Cushing's syndrome, the most common being iatrogenic (the use of exogenous steroids). However, the term 'Cushing's disease' is strictly used to describe Cushing's syndrome resulting from an ACTH-producing pituitary tumour or adenoma.

An overproduction of aldosterone from the zona glomerulosa of the adrenal cortex, as a result of a functioning adenoma, is known as Conn's syndrome. The overproduction of aldosterone leads to increased excretion of K^+ and H^+ from the distal convoluted tubule and collecting ducts of the kidney, resulting in a hypokalaemic metabolic alkalosis.

Endocrine physiology and thermoregulation – Answers

Adrenal insufficiency (also known as Addison's disease) results in decreased production of glucocorticoids and mineralocorticoids from the adrenal cortex. It is most commonly a result of destruction of the adrenal cortex by autoimmune adrenalitis. Decreased mineralocorticoid activity results in sodium loss and decreased potassium excretion, with consequent hyperkalaemia, hyponatraemia, volume depletion and hypotension. Hypoglycaemia may occasionally occur as a result of glucocorticoid deficiency and impaired gluconeogenesis. Stresses, such as infections, trauma or surgery, may precipitate a life-threatening adrenal crisis, which may prove fatal unless corticosteroid therapy is begun immediately.

Congenital adrenal hyperplasia (or adrenogenital syndrome) represents a group of autosomal recessive, inherited metabolic disorders characterised by a deficiency in a particular enzyme involved in the biosynthesis of cortical steroids, especially cortisol and aldosterone. 21-Hydroxylase deficiency accounts for 90% of cases. Steroidogenesis is then channelled into other pathways, leading to increased production of androgens, and virilisation in females and genital enlargement and/or precocious puberty in males. Simultaneously, the deficiency of cortisol results in increased secretion of ACTH, causing adrenal hyperplasia. Impaired aldosterone secretion leads to salt wasting. Patients are treated with exogenous steroids, which, in addition to providing adequate levels of glucocorticoids, suppress ACTH levels and thus decrease the synthesis of the steroid hormones responsible for many of the clinical abnormalities.

D Is essential for spermatogenesis

Testosterone is a steroid hormone, secreted by the interstitial cells (of Leydig) within the mature testis. It is essential for the growth and division of the germinal cells in forming sperm and in the development of the secondary sexual characteristics. Sertoli cells, on the other hand, are postulated to act as 'nurse' cells, providing structural and metabolic support for the developing spermatogenic cells.

Whereas FSH is trophic to Sertoli cells, LH is trophic to the Leydig cells. LH, secreted by the anterior pituitary, stimulates the Leydig cells to secrete testosterone through the formation of cAMP via the G-protein-coupled serpentine LH receptor. The secretion of LH in turn depends on the pulsatile release of GnRH from the hypothalamus. Androgen production from the adrenal cortex (and to a lesser extent from the ovaries) of females is normal and is responsible for the growth of pubic and axillary hair.

Oestrogen production during the menstrual cycle is principally 17β-estradiol. It increases steadily during the follicular phase to reach a peak before ovulation (when it has a positive feedback effect on the anterior pituitary, initiating the FSH and LH surges). Both FSH and LH are needed in order for ovulation to take place.

Fertilisation of the human ovum normally takes place in the outer third of the fallopian tubes. Over the next 5–7 days the fertilised ovum travels along the uterine tube and spends several days free in the uterus before implantation. This involves a complex series of events. A defect in any of the processes leading up to implantation may result in an abnormal extrauterine (or ectopic) pregnancy.

At the menopause, follicles disappear and are replaced by fibrous tissue. The decreased production of oestrogens from the ovaries results in loss of the negative feedback effect of oestrogens on the anterior pituitary and a rise in FSH. This rise in FSH can be measured and used to verify the start of the menopause.

Oestrogen production is mainly confined to ovarian tissue, but both the adrenal cortex and adipose tissue contribute to oestrogen production. Adipose tissue contains an aromatase enzyme that converts androgens to oestrogens. Oestrogen continues to be produced after the menopause and provides an ongoing stimulus for the formation of breast cancer. Tamoxifen blocks the action of oestrogen on breast tissue and is used in the treatment of breast cancer. Newer aromatase inhibitors block the peripheral conversion of androgens to progesterone. They are used to treat breast cancer in postmenopausal patients when oestrogen production from the ovaries ceases and where the peripheral conversion of androgens to oestrogens becomes more important.

Thermoregulation is one of the principal functions of the hypothalamus (not the thalamus). The central thermodetectors are located primarily within the preoptic area of the hypothalamus and to a lesser extent the adjacent areas of the anterior hypothalamus.

The apocrine sweat glands of the axilla, perineum and breast areolae have little role in thermoregulation. They are analogous to the odiferous glands of many mammals, but their biological significance in humans is unknown. It is the eccrine sweat glands that play an important role in heat loss by evaporation.

Non-shivering thermogenesis in brown fat is particularly important in keeping human infants and hibernating mammals warm. This process involves the uncoupling of oxidative phosphorylation within mitochondria via a specialised protein in the inner mitochondrial membrane called thermogenin. In adults, however, the importance of brown adipose tissue in heat generation is relatively small.

Humans are one of only a few animals who acclimate actively to heat. When exposed to hot weather for a period of 1–6 weeks, a person sweats progressively more profusely. This increased effectiveness of the sweating mechanism is caused by a direct increase in the sweating capability of the sweat glands themselves. Also associated with acclimatisation is a decrease in the concentration of sodium chloride in the sweat, which allows the conservation of body salt. Most of this effect is caused by increased secretion of aldosterone.

ANSWERS

Endocrine physiology and thermoregulation – Answers

Index

abducens nerve 16
acclimatisation 97
acenoids 17
achalasia 29
acid-base balance 106
ACTH 125
actin 76
action potential 75
Addison's disease 129
adrenal glands 46, 79
    disorders of 129
aldosterone 102
Allen's test 67
all or nothing law 75
altitude 97
amelia 3
anatomical snuffbox 60
angina pectoris 36
angiotensin I 103
angiotensin II 103, 107
angiotensin-converting enzyme 102
angiotensinogen 103
anterior spinal artery syndrome 25
antidiuretic hormone 105, 124
anti-Müllerian hormone 2
aortic opening 31
apoptosis 3
appendiceal mucocele 48
appendicitis 48
appendix, vermiform 47

aqueduct of Sylvius 71
arachnoid mater 23
arrhythmias 85
atherosclerosis 36
atrio-ventricular node 85
autonomic (involuntary) nervous system 79

baroreceptors 80, 90
Barrett's oesophagus 28
basilic vein 66
Bell's palsy 14, 18, 24
berry aneurysm 22
Berry's ligament 13
bile salts 117
birth, changes taking place at 1
bleeding 88
blood-gas barrier 98
Bohr shift 96
brachial plexus 62, 63
branchial cyst fistula 8
breast 26
Broca's area 70
Brodmann area 70
buccinator muscle 18, 19, 21
buccopharyngeal membrane 7
bursae 61

calcitonin 15
calcium
    in cardiac muscle 78
    metabolism 126

Calot's triangle 40
capillary hydrostatic pressure 89
caput medusae 43
carbaminohaemoglobin 95
carbon dioxide 95
carbon monoxide 98
carboxyhaemoglobin 95
cardiac muscle 36, 77
  calcium in 78
cardiac output 80
cardiovascular physiology 80
caroticocavernous fistula 20
carotid artery 19
carotid bodies 94
carpal tunnel 64
carpal tunnel syndrome 64
cauda equina 25
cavernous sinus 20
cebocephalia 6
cephalic vein 66
cerebral blood flow 90
cerebral cortex 70
cerebral perfusion pressure 90
cerebrospinal fluid 71
  constituents of 72
chemoreceptors 94
cholecystokinin 114
cholelithiasis 41
chorda tympani 14
Chvostek's sign 74
chylothorax 32
chymotrypsinogen 115
circle of Willis 22
cirrhosis 43
cleft lip/palate 6
clergyman's knee 61
Cloquet's lymph node 57

clotting cascade 88
clotting factors 88
congenital adrenal hyperplasia
  129
congenital diaphragmatic hernia
  5
conjunctiva 6
Conn's syndrome 129
Cooper's ligament 37
coronary arteries 36
coronary blood flow 84
cortisol 125
Courvoisier's law 41
cranial nerves 11
cretinism 127
cricoid cartilage 12
cricopharyngeus sphincter 29
cruciate ligaments 61
crura 31
cryptorchidism 2
culdocentesis 55
Cushing's reflex 90
Cushing's syndrome 125, 129
cyclopia 6

DeQuervain's tenovaginitis stenosans 60
diabetes insipidus 105
diabetes mellitus 109
  diagnosis 122
  type 1 121
diabetic ketoacidosis 128
diaphragm 5, 30
  innervation 30
diaphragma sellae 23
diplopia 16
ductus arteriosus 1

ductus venosus 1
Dupuytren's contracture 67
dura mater 23
dysphagia 29

electrocardiogram 81
emphysema 99
endarteritis obliterans 48
enophthalmos 16
enterokinase 115
epiglottis 12
epinephrine (adrenaline) 46
epiploic foramen of Winslow 38
Erb-Duchenne palsy 62
erythrocytes 86, 87
erythropoiesis 87
erythropoietin 44, 101
expiratory capacity 91
expiratory reserve volume 91
extradural haematoma 23
extraocular muscles 16

face, formation of 6
facial nerve 24
facial nerve palsy see Bell's palsy
Fahraeus-Lindqvist effect 87, 100
falciform ligament 1
falx cerebelli 23
falx cerebri 23
femoral artery 57, 65
femoral hernia 37
femoral triangle 57
fetal alcohol syndrome 6
fetal haemoglobin 96
Fick's law 98
field effect 50
follicle stimulating hormone 130
foramen of Magendie 71

foramen of Monro 71
foramen ovale 1
foramina of Luschka 71
fossa ovalis 1
Frank-Starling mechanism 78
Frank-Starling-Sarnoff mechanism 80
Frey syndrome 19
functional residual capacity 91

gallbladder 40
gallstones 41
gastric acid secretion 112
gastric mucosa 111
gastrin 113
gastrinoma 113
gastroepiploic arteries 49
gastro-oesophageal reflux disease 29
gastroschisis 7
genioglossus muscle 14
genital development 2
Gerota's fascia 42, 46
Glisson's capsule 42
glomerular filtration rate 108
glossopharyngeal nerve 14, 24
glucagon 116
gluconeogenesis 119
glucose
    absorption 118
    excretion 109
glycogenolysis 119
glycosuria 109
goblet cells 111
Goldblatt's hypertension 104
Goldman constant-field equation 75
goormaghtigh cells 104

greater (gastrocolic) omentum 49
Guillain-Barré syndrome 73
gut 7
Guthrie test 127
Guyon's canal 64

haemoglobin
  fetal 96
  formation of 100
haemoglobin-oxygen dissociation
  curve 96
haemorrhoids 54
haemostasis 88
haemothorax 32
Hagen-Poiseuille law 82
Haldane effect 95, 96
hand
  blood supply 67
  musculature 67
Harlequin syndrome 16
haustra 39
heart 36
hereditary spherocytosis 87
hernia 37
hiatus hernia 29
high-altitude sickness 97
Hilton's law 59
hip joint 59
Hirschsprung's disease 9
holoprosencephaly 6
hormones 124
Horner's syndrome 11, 16
housemaid's knee 61
hydrocele 2, 52
hydrocephalus 71
hypercalcaemia 15
hypercapnic response 94
hypertelorism 6

hyperventilation 97
hypoglossal nerve 14
hypothermia 84

iliofemoral ligament (of Bigelow)
  59
inguinal canal 37
inguinal hernia 2, 37
inspiratory capacity 91
inspiratory reserve volume 91
insulin 116, 123
  deficiency 128
intercostal neurovascular bundle
  27
interossei muscles 67
interstitial fluid
  colloid osmotic pressure 89
  hydrostatic pressure 89
intervertebral joints 25
intracerebral bleeding 23
intrinsic factor 111
islets of Langerhans 116

jaundice 41
jugulodigastric lymphadenopathy
  17
juxtaglomerular apparatus 104

Kehr's sign 40
keratitis 24
ketoacidosis 128
ketogenesis 119
kidney
  acid-base balance 106
  blood flow 107
  development 4
  glomerular filtration rate 108
Klinefelter syndrome 2

Index

Klumpke's palsy 62
knee joint 61
Kupffer cells 111
Kussmaul's breathing 128

Lacis cells 104
lactation 26
LaPlace's law 43, 80
large bowel 39
larynx 12
leptomeninges 23
levator palpebrae superioris 16, 24
Leydig cells 2
ligamentum arteriosum 1
ligamentum teres 1, 42
ligamentum venosum 1, 42
limb buds 3
limb development 3
lingual nerve 14
lingual thyroid 8
lipolysis 119
liver 117
liver capsule 42
loop of Henle 107
lower limb
    arterial supply 65
    venous drainage 66
lumbrical muscles 67
lungs 33
    capacities 91
    compliance 99
    gas exchange 98
    volumes 91
luteinizing hormone 130
lymph 89
lymphatic drainage
    breast 26

oesphagus 28
lymphatic trunk 32

McBurney's point 47
macula 68, 69
macula densa 104
main d'accoucheur 74
masseter muscle 21, 24
mastication, muscles of 21
Meckel's diverticulum 1, 10
meningitis 23
meningocele 9
menopause 131
menstrual cycle 131
mesonephric (wolffian) ducts 2
metanephric blastema 4
methaemoglobin 100
miosis 16
Monroe-Kelly doctrine 90
motor unit 74
mucosal rosette 29
Müller's muscle 16
mydriasis 11, 16
myelin sheath 73
myelomeningocele 9
myocardial oxygen demand 84
myoglobin 96
myosin 76

nasolacrimal duct 6
nasolacrimal groove 6
Nernst's potential 75
nerve conduction 73
nervi erigentes 54
nervous system 9
neural crest 9
neural tube 9
neuromuscular junction 79

neurulation 9
nitric oxide 83
nodes of Ranvier 73
norepinephrine (noradrenaline) 46, 79
nucleus accumbens 79

oblique fissure 33
oculomotor nerve 16
oedema 89
oesophageal opening 31
oesophagus 28
  constrictions 29
oestrogen 131
omental patch repair 49
omphalocele 7
optic chiasma 69
orbicularis oculi 24
osmoreceptors 105
ovaries 2, 53
oxytocin 124

pacemaker cells 85
palatine shelves 6
palatoglossal arch 17
palatoglossus muscle 14
palatopharyngeal arch 17
palmar aponeurosis 67
pampiniform plexus 52
pancreas 114
pancreatic enzymes 115
paramesonephric (müllerian) ducts 2
parathyroid adenoma 15
parathyroid glands 8, 15
parathyroid hormone 15, 126
parietal pleura 34
Parkinson's disease 79

parotid duct of Stensen 19
parotid gland 19, 110
pectoralis major 26
pelviureteric junction 50
pericardial fluid 35
pericardiocentesis 35
pericardium 35
peritoneal cavity, spaces 42
pes anserinus 19
pH 106
phaeochromocytoma 79
pharyngeal (branchial) arches 8
pharyngeal plexus 14
phocomelia 3
photoreceptors 69
phototransduction 68, 69
phrenic nerve 30
pia mater 22
pituitary gland 120
pituitary hormones 120, 124
plasma colloid osmotic pressure 89
plasmin 88
platelets 88
pleura 34
pleurisy 34
pleuroperitoneal membranes 5
pneumonia 34
popliteal artery 65
porsosystemic anastomoses 43
posterior cricoarytenoid muscles 12
pouch of Douglas 55
Poupart's ligament 37
Pringle's manoeuvre 38
Prinzmetal's angina 36
processus vaginalis 2
pterion 23

Index

pterygoid muscle 21, 24
ptosis 16
pulmonary blood supply 93
pulse pressure 93
Purkinje fibres 85

Ramsay Hunt syndrome 24
rectum 54
renin-angiotensin system 104
residual volume 91
retinitis pigmentosa 68
retromandibular vein 19
rhodopsin 68
rotator cuff 58
round ligament 51
rule of 2s 10
rule of thirds 18

saliva 110
salivary glands 110
salivary stones 19
saltatory conduction 73
saphenous veins 66
secretin 114
septum transversum 5
serratus anterior 62
Sertoli cells 2
sex chromosomes 2
shoulder joint 58
sialolithiasis 110
sickle cell anaemia 87
sick sinus syndrome 85
sino-atrial node 85
sliding filament theory 74
smooth muscle 76
sodium excretion 109
somatic (voluntary) nervous system 79

somatostatin 123
spermatic cord 51
sphincter of Oddi 117
spina bifida 9
spinal accessory nerve 18
spinal cord 25, 62
spinal nerves 11
spirometry 91
spleen 44
splenectomy 44
sppendices epiploicae 39
Starling's forces 89
starvation 119
stomach 7
    blood supply 56
    gastric acid secretion 112
    gastric mucosa 111
stylopharyngeus muscle 18
subarachnoid haematoma 23
subdural haematoma 23
superior laryngeal nerve 12
surfactant 92
sweat glands 132
syncope 80
syndrome of inappropriate ADH
    release 105

taeniae coli 39
tamoxifen 131
taste 14
temporalis muscle 21, 24
tentorium cerebelli 23
teratogens 3
testes 52
    descent of 2
testosterone 130
tetany 74
thalidomide 3

thermoregulation 132
thoracic duct 32
thyroglossal cyst 8
thyroid gland 8, 13, 127
thyroid stimulating hormone 13
thyroxine 127
tidal volume 91
tongue 8, 14
tonsillectomy 17
tonsils 17
total lung capacity 91
transpyloric plane (of Addison) 45
trapezius palsy 18
triiodothyronine 127
trochlear nerve 16
Trousseau's sign 74
trypsin 115
trypsin inhibitor 115
tuberculosis 34
tuftsin 44
Turner syndrome 2

umbilical arteries 1
upper limb, venous drainage 66
urachus (allantois) 1, 10
ureteric buds 4
ureters 50, 55
urothelium 50
uterus, supporting ligaments 55

valvulae conniventes 39
vasa recta 107
vascular response 83
vascular tone 11
vas deferens 51
vena cava opening 31
vertebral body 25
vesicoureteric junction 50
visceral pain 7
visceral pleura 34
visual cortex 68, 69
visual pathway 69
vitamin A deficiency 68
vitamin D 126
vitellointestinal duct 1, 10
vocal folds 12
Volkmann's ischaemic contracture
    67
volvulus 7

Waldeyer's ring 17
Wernicke's area 70
Wilms' tumour 4
WT-1 4

Zollinger-Ellison syndrome 113
zona fasciculata 46
zona glomerulosa 46
zona reticularis 46

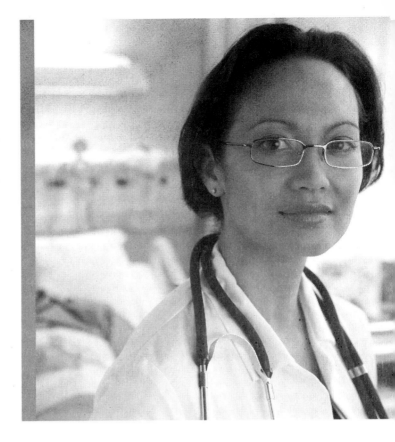

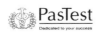
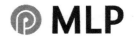